Body Stories

in and Out and WITH and through fAt

Edited by Jill Andrew and May Friedman

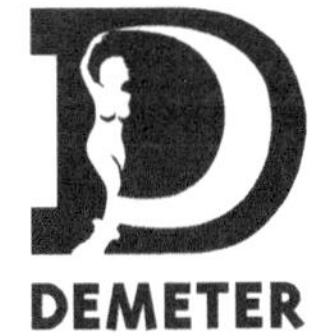

DEMETER

Body Stories

In and Out and With and Through Fat

Edited by Jill Andrew and May Friedman

Demeter Press
2546 10th Line
Bradford, Ontario
Canada, L3Z 3L3
Tel: 289-383-0134
Email: info@demeterpress.org
Website: www.demeterpress.org

Demeter Press logo based on the sculpture "Demeter" by Maria-Luise Bodirsky www.keramik-atelier.bodirsky.de

Printed and Bound in Canada

Cover design and typesetting: Michelle Pirovich

Library and Archives Canada Cataloguing in Publication
Title: Body stories: in and out and with and through fat /
edited by May Friedman and Jill Andrew.
Names: Friedman, May, 1975- editor. | Andrew, Jill, 1978- editor.
Description: Includes bibliographical references.
Identifiers: Canadiana 20200374664 | ISBN 9781772582543 (softcover)
Subjects: LCSH: Body image in women. | LCSH: Body image. | LCSH: Overweight women. | LCSH: Overweight persons. | LCSH: Overweight women, Psychology. | LCSH: Overweight persons, Psychology. | LCSH: Discrimination against overweight women. | LCSH: Discrimination against overweight persons. | LCSH: Obesity, Psychological aspects.
Classification: LCC BF697.5.B63 B63 2020 | DDC 306.4/613,Äîdc23

To all the contributors to this collection in its many iterations over the years who have laid bare their lived experience in and out and through fat and have shared their body stories

Acknowledgments

We begin by acknowledging that we live and work on Indigenous land, the traditional territory of many nations, including the Mississaugas of the Credit, the Anishnabeg, the Chippewa, the Haudenosaunee, and the Wendat peoples. We acknowledge that this land is now home to many diverse First Nations, Inuit, and Métis peoples. We strive to honour the land and to be here as respectful guests.

Body Stories: In and Out and With and Through Fat would not be here without our generous contributors past and present. Thank you for entrusting us with the power and vulnerability of your narratives. We hope as you move through these echoes of voices that you are able to see and feel our commitment to holding your stories with great care and reverence. *Body Stories* is the final iteration of *Phat Girls in Search of a Pretty World: Hot Lil' Fat Chicks Speakin' Out*—a project that began nearly two decades ago with the simple yet transformative goal of sharing women's stories about our bodies.

Jill: I want to extend my profound gratitude to the Ontario Arts Council for awarding me upon recommendations from Lois Pike at Sumach Press and Emily Schultz at Broken Pencil with 2003 Writer's Reserve grants. I can still remember the immense pride and validation I felt upon receiving the news. Thank you! Beth McAuley, our intermittent conversations and your guidance helped keep the oxygen going and the lights on. You supported me and my vision long before body positivity and fat activism caught the growing wind behind its back today.

To my friends and loved ones who have been around since the very beginning of this journey and to those I lost along the way, I will never forget your support. Relationships and interactions—our interconnectedness—plays such a significant role in each of our body stories. My dear Aisha, here we go again—another commitment completed, another finish line crossed! I couldn't have done any of it without you, your faith in my abilities and your consummate way of seeing me precisely at times when I struggle the hardest to see myself. Mom, you've raised a Black woman who won't stop talkin' back, takin' up space, and pushin' boundaries. I learned from the best!

Every independent bookstore, organization, small business, advocacy and arts collective, media outlet, online community, professor, students, feminists, and the countless colleges and universities that helped promote this project's calls for submissions—thank you. Nothing is accomplished in a vacuum. I'll never know all the names of those who helped me along the way. To our readers, I sincerely hope that you find a bit of yourself in these chapters, and if you don't, please let this inspire you to write your own because we can never have enough.

Last but certainly not least, Andrea O'Reilly, Demeter Press's publisher, and *Body Stories* coeditor May Friedman. You two. I fear my words could never be enough. Andrea, you saw the value in my project from day one and you stood firmly beside me. You connected me to May in the spring of 2014 and that began a beautiful relationship that sealed the fate of *Body Stories*. May and Andrea, thank you for your friendship and your collegial and editorial wit! I am also deeply thankful to your families for sharing you with me for all this time. We did it!

May: This project has been a labour of love and an epic journey. I wouldn't have made it to this point without the support of my friends and family, especially the sweet weirdos of Borden St. I also want to thank my colleagues at Ryerson University for helping to build a space where fat studies and fat activisms are beginning to gain recognition. Finally, my thanks to Jill for sharing her baby with me and trusting me to help bring this project to the world.

Contents

Introduction

Jill Andrew

"Halle Berry has a great laugh—it's full and rich, and she gets her whole body into it. It erupts as she's explaining why she still keeps a pair of Mickey Mouse blue jeans that she's had since she was 15. 'It's my annual test—I try them on once a year, and if I can still fit into them, then all is good in the world!' (Big surprise—she can)."—Tim Allis, interview with Halle Berry, *InStyle Magazine,* April 2007

"I'm fat but I don't want kittens and a country scene across the front of my shirt. I'd still like to get laid thank you very much."—Candy Palmater, from the documentary *Well Rounded,* 2020

This book is a labour of love and liberation. The project has followed twists and turns; it has resisted a smooth path in the same way that fat rolls and folds resist the imperative of leanness, of neat lines from here to there. Our bodies are messy, nonlinear; they often involve conflicting processes of being and becoming through our social interactions and intersectional subjectivities as well as through the materiality of our lives. I think about these ebbs and flows when I reflect on the unconventional trajectory of this project. The tremendous responsibility of holding people's stories twinned with my own vulnerability contributed to the many steps in the path to this book's arrival. But—let me start at the beginning.

I began this project in 2002. I saw a play called *The Adventures of a Black Girl in Search of God* written and produced by the award-winning Canadian playwright Djanet Sears. Themes in the play included race and representation, minstrels, and the racist and gendered stereotypes projected on to Black bodies. The play forced me to confront my own bodily uneasiness. I began to reflect on not only Black but also Black and fat embodiment. At the time I grappled with the unruliness of my body's Blackness and fatness even as I read and began to find community and pride in edited anthologies—such as *Turbo Chicks: Talking Young Feminisms, Shadow on a Tightrope: Writings by Women on Fat Oppression, Black Girl Talk, We're Rooted Here and They Can't Pull Us Up: Essays in African Canadian Women's History,* and *Naked: Black Women Bare All About Their Skin, Hair, Hips, Lips and Other Parts*—and the existence of local fat activist groups like Pretty Porky and Pissed Off as well as Fat Femme Mafia (FFM) and American non-profits like the fat-rights organization NAAFA (National Association to Advance Fat Acceptance).

I had been told so many times that I had "such a pretty face!" followed by the dreadful... "If you'd only..." Those voices took up space in my head, and I was tough on myself for not following the societal rules and was frustrated with my body for displaying my disobedience. As a young person, I would engage in unhealthy practices, such as yoyo dieting. Even after I began to read and study about weight discrimination and size activism as a young adult, I nonetheless remained enmeshed in my own struggles to not only accept but praise my body.

This project began as a way to talk to other women about how they felt about their bodies. I instinctively understood that to survive, I needed to create a space and a community where I didn't feel so alone. I saw that people around me needed this conversation too, even, or perhaps especially, when they seemed unable to have it.

As the idea grew in 2003 while a student at York University, I began to place flyers on telephone poles there and at other universities and colleges. I was also York University Excalibur newspaper's Special Issues: Women's Issues editorial coordinator that year which also helped me spread the word. I sent hundreds of emails and dropped off calls for submissions[1] at the Toronto Women's Bookstore and feminist sex shop Good for Her, among others. The initial lead title reflected my then discomfort with the word fat. Years before African American comedian and actress Mo'Nique would star in her 2006 film *Phat Girlz*, I called my project "Phat Girls in Search of a Pretty World: Hot Lil Fat Chicks Speakin' Out." "Phat" for me was then more about respectability than coolness. This term, in my opinion, obfuscated, hid, and apologized for fatness. Nonetheless, through the anthology, I sought to create that pretty world—to bring into existence the world I wished existed for me and other fat people. The book was about finding community and sharing voices with others and to work through our thoughts on ourselves.

Taking Up Space

Growing up I was often told "Jilly—good girls are seen and not heard." I became increasingly interested in understanding how fat people, especially women-identifying fat people, were living in a society that was hell bent on preventing us from taking up space and from being seen. I remember often being one of if not the tallest kid in the class. I was often read as older than I was, and I can still remember certain uncomfortable situations where I was adultified and oversexualized by men, who upon learning my age would appear shocked but would still inappropriately reference with an air of desire my "grown woman" body. I can still remember sucking in my stomach, trying to keep its jiggles from hanging over my jeans in pictures. Today, I look at many of these pictures, and I barely see a stomach. Perception's consequences can be tragic.

As I grew into adulthood, I wanted to reject that silencing and shrinking. I wanted to confidently take up space, to assert my fatness, and to come out in many different ways. This book was my way of insisting on holding my ground, on being both seen and heard. At the same time, trepidation got a hold on me. I felt the heavy responsibility of selecting people's stories for the anthology and for organizing people's experiences. At a certain point, I turned away. Life got busy, and I hid from the project, but I never forgot the stories I was walking with.

Years later, after growing older as well as into myself and my body politics, I knew the project couldn't remain unfinished. I refused to allow our stories to remain silent. I saw that the narrative around fatness wasn't changing—or if it was, it seemed at times worse. Social media illuminated growing fat activisms, body positivity movements, fatshion bloggers, and opportunities for self-valuation, but it also created space that some used to amplify hate and body injustice.

I began to work in schools in different roles from placement student, child and youth worker to teacher and student equity program advisor over the years and saw how everyday fat talk would manifest in playgrounds, in classrooms, in teachers talking about their failed diets, and in kids being berated in hallways by their peers, judgements flying based on what they ate or the clothing they wore. Fatness was stereotypically perceived as a character flaw and a sign of poor judgement, and, as such, it did not receive a passing grade. I saw some parents judged because of what their children did and did not eat. Inspiringly, I also saw teachers and caring adults actively working to reimagine the way children thought about their bodies and about fatness—a way that saw fat simply as another type of body, a description and not a prescription for hate, judgment, and social exclusion.

I reconnected with Dr. Andrea O'Reilly, who had been supportive of the project from its earliest years, and the project was reenergized. Andrea put me in touch with May, who had experience editing books and was writing and thinking about fatness and this latest version of the project was born. We began the project several years ago in between our busy lives, blending a mix of writing from the anthology's inception with newer chapters. I cannot say thank you enough to our contributors who stayed with this anthology through its iterations. Their stories have stood the test of time. I am also grateful to those who did not because their relationship with fatness had shifted or their voices had grown and manifested in other ways.

Body Stories

Fundamentally, this project is about owning our own stories. Body stories capture a more nuanced, interconnected, interactive, and complex telling of our understanding, perception, and experience of and through our body. Plenty has been published on body image, but image suggests a static fixed body unmitigated through our social interactions and varying times and spaces. Our project is not a "how-to" guide for fat confidence. It's not a compendium of fat suffering. It's simply a collection of body stories—narratives about what it's like to survive in a predominantly weight-hating world saturated by images and in a visual culture that levels significant social and cultural capital onto our skin. This project resists the ways that bodies marginalized are often written and researched about and the assumptions these misrepresentations can plant into people's idea about our existence.

The stories in this book are celebratory and are painful. Some are neutral. They look at intersections of race and queerness; they destabilize womanhood by presenting a range of possible feminized embodiments.

They explore issues of disability and madness. They grapple with popular culture, clothing, education, and the schooling of fat bodies. The project explores our bodies and healthcare. The project delves into intimacies, our intergenerational truths, and our body relationships at home, in our communities, and at work. This project explores our bodies through art, poetry, and the spoken word. I may not agree with every story, but the full range of possibilities that are collected here gives a picture of what it means to live in a society with strong and powerful messages about size, about normalcy, and about what a moral and healthy life and body look like. This book resists stability. It lays bare the nuances and complexities of fat and the ways in which many different truths and sizes can, and must, coexist.

Where We Are Now

When the book began, it was about finding out if I was the only person who was struggling. Since then, in innumerable ways, I have found that this is a universal struggle. Everyone is asking questions about weight, about being beautiful, about fitting in, and about the performances associated with all of these. These questions link to inquiries about our other identities and experiences. Somewhere along the way, I realized I had to borrow from the social model of disability (Garland Thomson) in that my body, our bodies, weren't the problem; the societal structures that constrained us were the problems, and it was here we needed to make change.

This message has never been clearer. We are all navigating through the grips of COVID-19, an unprecedented global pandemic. What we know from research is that this pandemic is already disproportionately affecting women, Black, Indigenous, people of colour, disabled and 2SLGBTQ+ communities. We have also seen in certain parts of the world that fat people, often written off early on by medical professions as bodies ravaged by so-called preexisting conditions, have had legitimate fears regarding access to ventilators and other life-saving procedures due to weight bias in care. This collection is coming to life at a historical moment, as now more than ever, it is crucial that fat and other bodies made marginalized and systemically threatened with erasure be reminded of our value and our right to human rights, equitable access and care.

The initial goal of this project was to collect stories, but the final work is to create the "pretty world" that I only dreamed of when the project began. This world would allow fat people to go to the doctor without fear. This world would have sartorial fabulousness in every size. This world would have space for fat bodies to fit in or fit out, and fitting out wouldn't automatically be a bad thing. And this world would help us unlearn damaging pedagogies and stifling categorizations of our bodies. I want this book to help create that world.

Into the Future

This book is a snapshot of its place and time, but these stories should remind us that we're here to stay. The body stories will change, but we will keep owning our own narratives. Although stories, especially those written by women, are often seen as outside the academic canon, I submit that these stories, these creative offerings, are theory, are research, and are activism. They are nothing less than the blueprint for liberation. Writing about fat and about bodies outside of medicalized narratives—without ignoring the effect of race, sexuality, class, ability, gender, fashion, appearance, and beyond—is radical and rigorous.

It is impossible to think about the future without wishing for liberation. Liberation can come in many forms. It can mean an awareness, the queering of knowledges, as well as the ability to name and confront. The stories in this book display the ways that liberation isn't necessarily a finish line or a thing we can complete; rather, it is a million actions and understandings in aid of a renewed and hopeful world, in which change for the better, especially for those furthest from the so-called centre, is the norm. This book is not to help create space for our bodies. We aren't asking for anything. It is to celebrate those who have already claimed the space our bodies deserve and to empower those still on the journey to stick with it.

I hope this book will serve anyone who is interested in digging into real stories about real people's journeys in and through and with their bodies. I hope that educators, students, scholars, activists, creatives and others will find wisdom in this book written over so many years of awakenings. I hope that the book adds to the stories that have influenced and inspired me and will hopefully provide inspiration, or at the very least aspiration, for the stories of the future.

Endnote

1. Although the language has changed from that of the original submissions, even then I was interested in an intersectional lens while documenting women's relationships, perceptions, and experiences through and with their bodies.

Works Cited

Bristow, Peggy, et al. *We're Rooted Here and They Can't Pull Us Up: Essays in African Canadian Women's History.* 2nd ed. University of Toronto Press, Scholarly Publishing Division, 1994.

Byrd, Ayana, and Akiba Solomon. *Naked: Black Women Bare All About Their Skin, Hair, Hips, Lips and Other Parts.* TarcherPerigee, 2005.

Garland Thomson, Rosemarie. "Misfits: A Feminist Materialist Disability Concept." *Hypatia: A Journal of Feminist Philosophy,* vol. 26, no. 3, 2001, pp. 591-609.

Mitchell, Allyson, Lisa Bryn Rundle, and Lara Karaian. *Turbo Chicks: Talking Young Feminisms* (Women's Issues Publishing Program). Sumach Press, 2001.

Schoenfielder, Lisa, and Barb Wieser. *Shadow on a Tightrope: Writings by Women on Fat Oppression.* Aunt Lute Books, 1983.

The Black Girls. *Black Girl Talk.* Sister Vision: Black Women and Women of Colour Press, 1995.

Well Rounded. Directed by Shana Myara, Canadian Filmmakers Distribution Centre (CFMDC), 2020.

1.

Because I'm Fat, I Don't Deserve Satisfaction? A Young Fat Woman's Experience of Sex

Samantha Keene

On Friday or Saturday nights in my town, the aim of the game is to hook up. These casual sexual relations generally occur after consuming alcohol, socializing, and flirting in bars. One night, it's 4:00 a.m. The lights have gone from dim to bright and are scorching the bloodshot eyes of the night's revellers. The DJ spins a song about nobody going home alone. As I search for familiar faces, I feel a tap on my shoulder. I turn around, expecting to see my friends. Instead, a man I have not met asks my plans for the night. I tell him I am shortly heading home. He looks me up and down, slowly, his eyes scouring every inch of my ample body. He traces my body outline twice, before saying "You'll do."

Hold on. I'll do? What does that even mean? Am I what is left for the taking? The easy option for a casual lay? Am I supposed to settle for someone who thinks that I'll do?

To be fat is to be different, and although there are different levels or conceptions of what fat is, the word alone carries negative connotations. To be fat is to be weak, lazy, undesirable, and definitely not sexually confident. I am the opposite of these descriptors. I am a young, single, Pākehā woman living in Wellington, New Zealand. I am a PhD student studying pornography and sex, and I am also a woman of size. I have an active social life, and I am confident in my own sexuality. This chapter discusses the way that (hetero)sexual experiences occur in a climate where fat women are considered deviant as they contravene dominant Western beauty ideals that view thinness as attractive. Furthermore, this chapter provides my own personal voice in a space where there is sparse academic literature on fat women's sexual experiences, as "most of the research has concentrated on perceivers' opinions about fat persons' sexuality, or men's exploitative sexual experiences with fat women as "hoggers"[1] or fat admirers" (J. A. Gailey, *Transforming,* 55). Although my experiences are not intended to be generalizable and are in many ways inherently personal and occur within a particular social context, I believe that some of these experiences are reflective of other fat women's experiences. These experiences may be common to other fat women due to the degrees of fatphobia in society and the way that fat women who are agentic in their sexuality are perceived as deviant. First, I discuss fat women as easy targets and highlight how this assumption has manifested in my experiences with men to date. Second, I explore the way that I have experienced a silence about men having sex with a fat woman, as such a liaison may be embarrassing for men to engage in. Lastly, I discuss the ways that I believe mainstream pornography perpetuates stereotypes about fat sex and presents it as a niche area that fetishizes fat bodies.

Fat Women as Easy Targets

Media representations of sex for people in their twenties and living a similar student lifestyle demonstrate a permissive sexuality, which incorporates frequent casual sex, with decreased emphasis on committed relationships (Garcia et al.). Living in this hook-up culture means that although not everyone is "hooking up", the pressure to be part of that culture certainly prevails. And while that pressure might be felt by all people regardless of size, for me, being a fat woman in a hook-up culture feels almost paradoxical. On the one hand, the pressure to engage in a hook-up culture is ever present. On the other, engaging in that hook-up culture contravenes societal and cultural understandings of what it is to be a fat woman, which is seldom seen as sexy (J. Gailey, *Hyper*).

J. Gailey *Hyper* contends that fat women occupy a space in society where they are simultaneously hypersexual and nonsexual, and it's this type of dichotomous thinking that I have encountered in my sexual interactions. In one way, I am expected to be this sexually insatiable being, so desperate for affection that I will take whatever is on offer. Michael Flood contends that men codify particular sayings such as "fat chicks need lovin' too" (347) to signify the ways that they circumvent the flirting and wooing process needed in the sexual marketplace with conventionally attractive women. As fat women are not seen as conventionally attractive, such women are therefore a so-called easier option to have sex with (Gailey and Prohaska). It is this kind of thinking that helps me make sense of that phrase "you'll do" I referred to earlier. For the man that night, I was a sure bet. I would be unlikely to say no. As a fat woman, I'm certainly not having frequent sex, so surely I would jump at the opportunity to have sex with him, right?

He could not be more wrong, which suggests a paradox. As a young fat woman, I am also viewed as sexually deviant for engaging in the hook-up culture because to be fat and sexually confident is implausible in the eyes of others. On the occasions that I have hooked-up—in the same way that my thin friends do—it becomes a group discussion point, and my sexual encounters are dissected because they are viewed as outside the norm, in a way that others are not. Being fat and getting laid seems extraordinary. In fact, it was only six months ago that this became clear for me. I had met someone online who came out for a night on the town with my friends. He was, as everyone noticed, conventionally attractive. During the night, he was holding my hand under the table. Everyone's eyes were locked on us. He kissed me in front of everyone, and it was this public display of affection that saw the whole table erupt. All my friends clapped, hooted, and made a scene out of his display. I was mortified. I had never seen such a response to someone getting kissed. Would this have happened if he was not conventionally attractive? I doubted it, as me settling for someone who is not conventionally attractive is expected of fat women. The next day, I was expected to provide a rundown of the evening's later events, as if my involvement with an attractive man was an issue of public concern and fascination. It was the public and overt display of my sexual availability and desirability that was key here, as it violated the expected norms of fat women as unsexy, as undesirable, and as only prepared to settle with other nonconventionally attractive people.

The Hidden Nature of Hooking Up with a Fat Woman

The extraordinariness of fat sexual desirability discussed earlier is also present in how men talk about the sex they have with fat women and the interaction between relationships, size, and traditional, heterosexist masculinities. These themes were made evident in an experience I had with a man I recently met. We had chatted earlier and exchanged phone numbers. He met me at a bar a block and a half from my house and suggested we get a taxi and head home. I mentioned how close by I lived, and that it made more sense to walk, but he insisted. I queried his persistence, why was a taxi trip so important? It was then he told me he was concerned that his friends would spot him taking home a fat chick. I could not believe it!

J. Gailey's chapter on ample sex describes the ways that men who have sex with fat women often do not identify as exclusively interested in them, and many who are "genuinely attracted to women of size may keep it a secret to avoid reprisal" (*Hyper* 114). The same can be said for men that are taking home a fat girl for an "easy" lay or to break a dry spell. In fact, such sexual encounters may be shrouded in secrecy, as having sex with a fat woman, especially if he continues to see her, may encourage a man to be judged by his peers (Flood).

Although some heterosexual encounters with fat women may result in public secrecy about private intimacy, the pervasiveness of fat shame may also shut down private sexual moments. This theme of approach-avoidance was evident with another man I recently encountered, who, when we were out together, was very publicly affectionate, almost to the extent that it was over the top. At home, he was the opposite. He struggled to be sexually interested because he had "never been with a fat girl" and did not want his friends finding out because it was not the "done thing" or "manly," even though he had feelings for me. Hearing that hurt. Not only was it offensive to me, but it also showed how toxic stereotypes about fat women and their bodies are. Clearly, engaging in sexual relations with a fat woman would see these men lose masculinity status points. In this way, then, such secrecy about fat sex may serve to perpetuate the hypersexual-nonsexual divide alluded to earlier, as it silences discussions about the realities of fat sex, thus increasing assumptions about fat women as nonsexual. Simultaneously, however, it also has the potential for hypersexualizing fat sex by increasing its excitement and entertainment value as a silent and secret act.

Fat in Pornography

Mainstream heterosexual pornography displays a particular aesthetic that appeals to a narrow trope of cultural beauty ideals (Mattebo et al.), which depict thinness as attractive. It's no surprise then that the average pornography actress is on the slender side. In 2009, *Adult Video News* released its first issue featuring a big, beautiful woman (BBW) alongside a discussion of the BBW industry. Goda Klumbyte and Katrine Smiet saw this publication as "a signal that pornography featuring fat female bodies is no longer an anomaly, but has reached a mainstream position in the adult entertainment landscape" (125). However, Michael Goddard describes the development of BBW pornography as facilitated by digital media networks that have created niche industries for this type of material. April Flores, a plus-sized pornography performer, notes that much BBW pornography "crosses into not so thinly veiled degradation and shame ... it's implied that viewers who like to watch us are freaks, too" (280). A male friend of mine invited me into his room one day and asked me what I thought about a pornographic clip he was watching. It was a BBW performer, and he talked about how it was a novel discovery for him. He liked the way that she "took it like a champ," but he felt guilty for watching it. I queried the guilt, to which he responded that fat pornography is the type of thing that you watch, but you do not want to enjoy because it is so out there and different.

Does that mean that men feel guilty for having sex with me? Am I really that different? I believe that the couching of BBW pornography as a kink or niche category contributes to these sorts of beliefs, and it also makes me feel that the type of sex I have, as a woman of size, is marginal and different to the mainstream. Although many people may feel empowered through watching BBW pornography (Klumbyte and Smiet), when BBW pornography continues to portray fat sex as something that freaks watch, or has freaks in them, I cannot help but feel that such representations inevitably contribute to the stereotypes about fat women and sex.

So, what does this all mean, then? Well, it's hard being a fat woman who is confident in her sexuality, as the "mainstream media's representations and discussions around sex makes it clear that fat people are not considered sexually attractive, or as individuals with sexual agency" (Pausé 43). But such views do not mean that fat women should have to settle in their sexual decision-making. Some men entertain the idea that fat women are easy sexual targets, and societal views determine the way fat sex is understood, which is undoubtedly exacerbated by framing fat pornography as freaky or somehow worthy of degradation and humiliation. However, fat women can be agentic in their sexuality.

Living in a hook-up culture is tough, and the pressures on women, especially fat women, to participate may come at an unreasonably high cost. Women around the world run the risk of experiencing the depressing realities of sexual double standards for male and female sexuality, whereby partaking in a hook-up culture labels men "studs" and women "sluts." But it's realizing these pressures, and understanding what makes them, that has made me who I am today: a confident, sexually agentic woman who refuses to view herself as sexually naive, as sexually desperate, or as only available for other's entertainment. The woman that I am today, and the confidence I have in myself, is a result of overcoming these barriers, and I am not defined by my size. I now know, through my experiences of unsexy sex, that I am sexy, worthy of satisFAcTion, and that there is no need for me to settle.

Endnotes

1. "Hoggers" refers to men who "prey on overweight or unattractive women to satisfy their competitive and/or sexual urges" (Gailey and Prohaska 32).

Works Cited

Flood, Michael. "Men, Sex, and Homosociality: How Bonds between Men Shape Their Sexual Relations with Women." *Men and Masculinities*, vol. 10, no. 3, 2008, pp. 339-59.

Flores, April. "Being Fatty D: Size, Beauty, and Embodiment in the Adult Industry." *The Feminist Porn Book: The Politics of Producing Pleasure*, edited by Tristain Taormino et al., The Feminist Press, 2013, pp. 279-83.

Gailey, Jeannine. *The Hyper(in)Visible Fat Woman: Weight and Gender Discourse in Contemporary Society*. Palgrave Macmillan, 2014.

Gailey, Jeannine A. "Transforming the Looking-Glass: Fat Women's Sexual Empowerment through Body Acceptance." *Fat Sex: New*

Directions in Theory and Activism, edited by Helen Hester and Caroline Walters, Routledge, 2016, pp. 51-66.

Gailey, Jeannine A., and Ariane Prohaska. ""Knocking Off a Fat Girl": An Exploration of Hogging, Male Sexuality, and Neutralizations." *Deviant Behavior*, vol. 27, no. 1, 2006, pp. 31-49.

Garcia, Justin R., et al. "Sexual Hookup Culture: A Review." *Review of General Psychology: Journal of Division 1 of the American Psychological Association*, vol. 16, no. 2, 2012, pp. 161-76.

Goddard, Michael. "Techno-Archaism, Excessive Corporeality and Network Sexuality." *C'lick Me: A Netporn Studies Reader*, edited by Katrien Jacobs, Marije Janssen, and Matteo Pasquinelli, Institute of Network Cultures, 2011, pp. 187-96.

Klumbyte, Goda, and Katrine Smiet. "Bodies Like Our Own? The Dynamics of Distance and Closeness in Online Fat Porn." *Fat Sex: New Directions in Theory and Activism*, edited by Helen Hester and Caroline Walters, Routledge, 2016, pp. 125-40.

Mattebo, Magdalena, et al. "Hercules and Barbie? Reflections on the Influence of Pornography and Its Spread in the Media and Society in Groups of Adolescents in Sweden." *The European Journal of Contraception, Reproductive Health Care*, vol. 17, no. 1, 2012, pp. 40-49.

Pausé, Cat. "Human Nature: On Fat Sexual Identity and Agency." *Fat Sex: New Directions in Theory and Activism*, edited by Helen Hester and Caroline Walters, Routledge, 2016, pp. 43-53.

2.

"Neither Sari nor Sorry": An Open Letter to the Indian Yummy Mummy

Sucharita Sarkar

Dear Indian Yummy Mummy,

I am writing to you from my oppositional subject position as a "tummy mummy," and I will attempt here to understand and interrogate the discourse of maternal bodies wherein you and I are situated. Yes, "tummy mummy" is the name my daughters have given me, more in loving observation than in sneering derision. I do not fit into the contours of the standardized yummy mummy, and I carry on my body the marks of "reproductive activity—stretch marks, breasts that have nursed, and postpartum weight" (Wolf 226), even a decade after giving birth.

Let me begin by acknowledging the transgressive potential of your self-focused identity project. You have interrupted the traditional discourse of good Indian motherhood, which valorizes selfless service, and have reclaimed your body as a site of agentic transformation.

Indian mothers have been culturally expected to be plump. The new mother almost always stays in her natal home, where her own mother and other female relations insist on "the unusually nutritious and fattening diet, and the compulsory rest for at least five weeks" (Kosambi 135). This practice is intended to ensure a steady supply of breastmilk, and the concomitant weight gain is disregarded, since the primary role of the new mother is to breastfeed her child and not to focus on herself. Although Indian mothers may benefit from the support offered in this postnatal stage, the construction of the maternal body as now predominantly serving as a tool for the sustenance of another also inevitably desexualizes the mother. This devoted, de-eroticized mother is always visually represented as draped modestly in a sari. This "strip of unstitched cloth four to nine metres in length" has an "ancient heritage associated with tradition and so-called feminine virtues like shame, introversion, decorum and respectability" (Sarkar 278). Especially after the sari was reformed during the Victorian colonial period—with the addition of the culturally borrowed blouse and petticoat—it became an ideal garment to camouflage large bodies and to shield sexualized bodies from public view. Sari-covered, fat maternal bodies became visible markers of class and caste status. However, the moral policing of the maternal bodily appearance betrayed a lack of concern for maternal agency and prioritized children's wellness over maternal physical and mental health (Kosambi 142). The ideal of maternal self-sacrifice was in practice a code for self-neglect, and mothers wholly dedicated to the service of the family rarely found time to take care of themselves.

As a working mother with two daughters, I reject the sari as a garment of daily wear. Not only is this my everyday symbolic resistance to the sari's problematic and gendered history, it is also a corporeal protest: the sari restricts my gait. Despite the advice of style experts that plus-sized Indian bodies look good in saris, I do not wear them. So, I applaud you, yummy mummy, when you, too, reject the sari. You would rather look fabulous in a "Diane von Furstenberg wrap dress" (George 136). You have rejected the stereotype of the middle-class and upper-caste Hindu Indian mother as a plump, sari-clad matron, happy in her role as cook and caregiver to her multigenerational, extended family. When a self-defined yummy mummy like actor Karisma Kapoor affirms, "I won't stop focusing on myself. I will take time out to fix myself for myself," I celebrate her refusal to neglect herself (Kapoor 132). Theoretically, I accept the poststructuralist feminist possibility that women's "body work, whether through exercise, cosmetics, or plastic surgery, can function as a meaningful source of empowerment" (Johnston and Taylor 945). I applaud you for resexualizing the mother and for bridging the gap between maternity and sexuality, a gap so long concealed in the nine-yard folds of the sari.

Yummy mummy, establishing the validity of your self-directed desires has not been easy for you. Media reports question your relevance in the Indian context, accuse you of wasting money and time at "gyms, slimming centres, liposuction options," and compare you negatively with the earlier generation of mothers who are "plump" and do not "wear sleeveless clothes" or makeup but who are, instead, "clued in about her children's whereabouts, her husband's work, [and who] look after the elderly" (Press Trust of India). Whereas fat, covered-up maternal bodies are approved as docile, your self-loving, sexualised, and disruptive body provokes moral panic and outrage.

However, yummy mummy, that is not the only response that you generate. Celebrity yummy mummies generate complex and often contradictory reactions in noncelebrity mothers—from envy, to mimicry, to inspiration, and to desperation and depression. I, too, have a contrarian complex of responses to you. Allow me to explore these responses.

Celebrity yummy mummies reiterate that the fat maternal body signifies a loss of selfhood and, indeed, that fat bodies are inherently deviant and problematic. Actor Sonali Bendre Behl recalls the time when her prepregnancy clothes did not fit her and writes, "I felt lost. It was as if I was living in someone else's body.... I was a complete mess" (Bendre Behl 21). In a lifestyle magazine interview that projected her as "mommylicious," actor Shilpa Shetty Kundra says: "I was as fat as a cow. I was a size 14 for the first time in my life! It made me feel strange because it didn't feel like me—and I just wanted to be me" (qtd. in Dadyburjor 77). As the monstrous, obese body becomes disciplined and, literally, reshaped into acceptable trim parameters, the yummy mummy expresses her elation at this transformation: "You begin to feel like a woman again, not just a mother whose sole responsibility is to raise her children" (George 55). Hence, the reclaiming of the body becomes an act of reclaiming a selfhood beyond motherhood. Fitness enthusiast Naomi George urges, "It is time for a little self-loving, time to reclaim the woman within" (143). I agree that this decision to reprioritize self-love is persuasive and liberating. I endorse the privileging of maternal fitness and health.

Yet, yummy mummy, I want to interrogate the notion of selfhood that you celebrate. Karisma Kapoor shares "the most important tip to lose weight": keep looking at "before-and-after pictures of yourself," which will "inspire" you to eat less and exercise more (102). This is how self-shaming of the fat body underpins the transformative self-love project of the yummy mummy. Blogger-author Kiran Manral writes of her "abdomen after childbirth": "Imagine a hot-air balloon collapsed and lying on a mucky field.... Who would want to make love to that? That is how *every* new mom feels when she ... looks at her body post childbirth" (my emphasis, 32). Here, she is reviling the fat body as "asexual, out of control" and physically and "morally repugnant" (Johnston and Taylor 945). The obverse of the yummy mummy's self-reclamation is a history of self-directed fatphobia, sexual anxiety, and objectification of the body.

Yes, yummy mummy, your project to perfect your body and reclaim your self is impelled by your internalized patriarchal cultural codes that devalue the female self and commoditize the female body. By rejecting and loathing your own past maternal fatness, you comply with the false binary between maternity and sexuality that is enforced by hetero-patriarchy to control the reproductive agency of mothers.

This self-hate is echoed even by mothers whose lives are not scrutinized by the media. For instance, the anonymous blogger sharing her weight loss story on *Mommy's Wall* writes, "Once I delivered my baby, everyone I met was like 'OMG you have gained so much weight.' I hated it. I was obese and heavy.... I was getting depressed with my over-sized clothes. I hated looking at myself in the mirror" (Admin para 1-3). Most Indian mom blogs have separate sections on weight loss, in which similar stories of self-punishing fatphobia are shared and circulated.

Blogger Sangeetha Menon, in her homepage at *Bumps n Baby*, reveals that she spends her time "asking her hubby if she is fat for the 'n'th time" (Menon). Kundra also emphasizes the continuous effort required: one has to "keep at it" (qtd. in Dadyburjor 77). The yummy mummy body project conceals a deep performance anxiety: it is always a becoming rather than a being, as it entails continual monitoring of boundaries and controlling of appetites. To use Judith Butler's terms, the yummy mummy can be regarded as a "repeated stylization of the body, a set of repeated acts within a highly rigid regulatory framework" (45).

Yummy mummy, this framework is apparently of your own choosing, yet your choice is overdetermined by "the hegemonic ideology of gendered beauty" (Johnston and Taylor 954). Your self-hate is caused by a misrecognition, and it is often exacerbated by the mirror, which functions as a metaphor for the gaze of others. Even as you decide to transform your postpartum fatness into yummy mummy fitness, you are the Foucauldian "docile body"—"subjected, used, transformed and improved" (Foucault 136), according to the dominant global-patriarchal beauty standards. The annual yummy mummy survey conducted by research agency AC Nielsen across urban centres in India reports that "92% of expecting fathers want their wives to be Yummy Mummy post their pregnancies ...[with] the same pre pregnancy bodies" (qtd. in Das para 2). Yet, yummy mummy, you insist that slimness and beauty are prerequisites of your selfhood and self-acceptance, and this insistence legitimizes the coercive notion that every modern Indian mother should become a yummy mummy to attain self-worth.

Yummy mummy, your antecedents can be traced to the post-1991 "new Indian woman" (1991 was when the government's new economic policy introduced neoliberalism to the nation). Rupal Oza describes this middle-class, upper-caste, and "rich and fashionable" woman as the "mimetic trope of the nation in globalization" (13). Your neoliberal individualism is not merely an unequivocal import or imitation of Western norms of maternal beauty; it is hybridized with Indian moral codes. Kundra balances global standards of beauty with local traditions of health, when she urges us to adopt "the Great *Indian* Diet" and "techniques and tips," such as yoga and meditation, which "are part of *Indian* history" (my emphasis, Kundra and Coutinho 169). Karisma Kapoor advises Indian yummy mummies to reject the unbridled consumerism and competitiveness of "Hollywood celebrity moms" in favour of Indian values of financial prudence (176). Both Kundra and Kapoor reveal an anxiety about the corrupting influences of the West, and a need to be modern (read "Western") but rooted in Indian traditions. Yet, yummy mummy, your engagement with these contradictory discourses of globalization and nationalism is celebratory rather than critical. You conflate the two discourses without questioning the disjunctures within this Indian-Western construct. I do not want the differences between us as individuals, or between discrete value systems, to be uncritically absorbed into the globalized flows of desire and consumption. I would rather politicize this difference and emphasize my alterity to resist the homogenizing tendencies of the neoliberalism that you embody.

The media-circulated visual-textual narratives of celebrity yummy mummies have created a globalized culture of celebrity worship and imitation. These images of magically swift postdelivery erasure of celebrity maternal fatness seduce not yet yummy mummies to opt for surgical interventions, such as mommy makeovers. The cosmetic surgery industry in India thrives on the insecurity of fat bodies and the promise of instant metamorphoses. The website of *Allure Med Spa* promises that their mommy makeover procedures—which address "post-pregnancy body issues in a *single-session* surgery," which includes a tummy tuck, breast lift, liposuction, and labiaplasty—will "leave *him* breathless" (my emphasis, Doshi para 2). This surgery narrative emphasizes the male gaze and exploits the feminine anxiety that seeks its approval. I choose not to offer my body as a surgically perfected commodity for the consumption of others. I choose not to mutilate my natural, whole body—fat or not—into "two-thirds of the women we could be" (Wolf 232).

Among Indian yummy mummies, though, mommy makeover surgery is an invisible, socially stigmatized, and secret stratagem of body control. Most celebrity mothers publicly endorse only natural methods, such as diet and exercise. When Shilpa Shetty Kundra encourages us mothers to shift our perspective from "weight loss" to "fat loss," she seems to replace the exclusionary antifat discourse with an inclusive, prohealth lifestyle discourse: "Shift your focus from the [weighing] scale to being consistent with your food, exercise, sleep and emotional health, and fat loss will surely follow" (Kundra and Countinho 122). Karisma Kapoor's yummy mummy guide acknowledges the differences in maternal bodies: "It depends on each person and each pregnancy.... Decide for yourself what and how much is right" (98).

Yet she does not allow for the continued or guilt-free existence of deviant fat bodies and declares, "There is no excuse for not looking after yourself" (Kapoor 98). Her guidebook polices fat bodies, and the size acceptance is only temporary, for the first few months after birth. When Shilpa Shetty Kundra writes, "Weight and discipline are [inversely] proportional to each other," she is also stigmatizing fat bodies as undisciplined and unruly (Kundra and Countinho 105). Under the superficial guise of body inclusiveness and consciousness raising, this fat shaming forecloses feminist maternal community building and positions fat mothers as unacceptable.

Yummy mummy, I retaliate by not accepting your reiterative linking of fat bodies to both disease and dis-ease. Kundra writes of her postpartum body which was heavier by "32 kilos": "I wanted my body back really badly, not just for the sake of looks, but because I *felt unhealthy*. I *did not feel my natural self* on the inside or the outside" (my emphasis, Kundra and Countinho, Preface x). In such statements, I read a disaffected horror of the fat self, which is deliberately marked as unnatural and, thus, unhealthy. Through a slippage of meaning, fitness and health—supposedly an integration of the physiological and the psychological—are reduced to the notion of slimness, which, when achieved, will produce a sense of satisfaction and self-confidence. I reject this distorted definition of health as a calibrated slimness that indicts all fat mothers as unhealthy and incapable of self-confidence. Simultaneously, I also question the media blaming of fat Indian mommies for raising fatty kids by being bad role models who prefer to dine out on unhealthy junk food rather than cook healthy, balanced meals: why does this survey conducted by the National Diabetes, Obesity, and Cholesterol Foundation demonize fat children, render Indian fathers (especially fat ones) irrelevant, and reassert that childcare is primarily the duty of the good mother? (Chaudhry para 1).

Faced by such biases, I understand that the yummy mummy is a potential space for mothers' identity formation beyond the stereotypes of good motherhood, a site that can, and often does, celebrate one's sexuality, self-worth, and empowerment. Yet the necessity of confining oneself to dominant norms of femininity, despite the lure of public approval and peer acceptance, is restrictive to me. Yummy mummy, you openly defy the pervasive ideology of self-sacrificing good Indian motherhood, yet your counter-cultural alterity itself becomes a hegemonic discourse that excludes fat mothers, not to mention other nonnormative mothers, such as mothers with disabilities, queer mothers, and many others. You do not radically challenge the institution of motherhood; you merely replace one coercive construct (the sacrificing mother) with another (the slim mother).

In opposition to your disciplined, slimmed body, I flaunt my deviant, fat one—a body that is part of, but does not wholly constitute or consume, my selfhood. I affirm that despite my "big stomach on which [I] focus," I am "nevertheless more than just a big stomach" (Orbach 113). Yes, I admit to residual, intermittent feelings of envy, regret, and inadequacy, but my corporeal experience of fatness will not make me negate your significance or agentic potential. I am engaging in a "new relationship with my body," choosing to refuse "self-loathing" for a "more accepting attitude" towards myself (Orbach 238-40). Yummy mummy, by deconstructing you, I wish to make space for the multiplicity of maternal bodies that exist between the sari and size zero—to make space for my own body and other maternal bodies that are both like and unlike mine and yours.

I belong to this intermediate space between our sari-wrapped, self-denying mothers and self-fashioning, size-obsessed yummy mummies, like you. I will engage with my body at my own pace and on my own terms.

Differentially yours,
Tummy Mummy

Works Cited

Admin. "Fastest and Most Efficient Weightloss for Obese People and My Inspiration." *Mommy's Wall*, www.mommyswall.com/fastest-efficient-weightloss-obese-people-inspiration. Accessed 12 Apr. 2016.

Bendre Behl, Sonali. *The Modern Gurukul: My Experiments with Parenting*. Random House India, 2015.

Butler, Judith. *Gender Trouble: Feminism and the Subversion of Identity*. Routledge, 1990.

Chaudhry, Lakshmi. "Fat Indian Mommy: Perfect Scapegoat for Child Obesity." *Firstpost*, www.firstpost.com/living/the-fat-indian-mommy-the-perfect-scapegoat-for-child-obesity-827453.html. Accessed 14 Apr. 2016.

Dadyburjor, Farhad. J. "Lights...Camera...Motherhood." *HiBlitz*, January 2014, pp. 70-81.

Das, Purba. "Indian to-Be Fathers Want Their Wives to Be Seen as 'Yummy Mummies'! What Does That Say of Indian Men?" *Business Insider*, www.businessinsider.in/indian-to-be-fathers-want-their-wives-to-be-seenas-yummy-mummies-what-does-that-say-of-indian-men/articleshow/47176950.cms. Accessed 12 Apr. 2016.

Doshi, Paresh. "Become a Yummy Mummy with Mommy Makeover Procedure." *Mommy Makeover India*, www.mommymakeoverindia.com/become-a-yummy-mummy-with-mommy-makeover-procedure/. Accessed 1 May 2016.

Foucault, Michel. *Discipline and Punish: The Birth of the Prison*. Translated by Alan Sheridan. Penguin, 1977.

George, Naomi. *Mum-Me: How I Raised Babies, Survived Toddlers and Learnt to Love Myself*. Harper Collins Publishers, 2014.

Johnston, Josee, and Judith Taylor. "Feminist Consumerism and Fat Activists: A Comparative Study of Grassroots Activism and the Dove Real Beauty Campaign." *Signs*, vol. 33, no. 4, 2008, pp. 941-66.

Kapoor, Karisma. *My Yummy Mummy Guide: From Getting Pregnant to Being a Successful Working Mom and Beyond*. Penguin, 2013.

Kosambi, Meera. *Crossing Thresholds: Feminist Essays in Social History*. New Delhi: Permanent Black, 2007.

Kundra, Shilpa Shetty and Luke Countinho. *The Great Indian Diet: Busting the Fat Myth*. Random House India, 2015.

Manral, Kiran. *Karmic Kids: The Story of Parenting Nobody Told You!* Hay House Publishers India, 2015.

Menon, Sangeetha. "About Me." *Bumps n Baby*, www.bumpsnbaby.com/about-me/. Accessed 12 Apr. 2016.

Orbach, Susie. *Fat Is a Feminist Issue*. Arrow Books, 1978.

Oza, Rupal. *The Making of Neoliberal India: Nationalism, Gender and the Paradoxes of Globalization*. Routledge, 2006.

Press Trust of India. "How Relevant is Yummy Mummy Title for Young Indian Moms?" *India TV*, www.indiatvnews.com/lifestyle/news/are-young-indian-moms-are-yummy-mummy-2557.html. Accessed 12 Apr. 2016.

Sarkar, Mahua. "Cultural Construction of Gender in Colonial Bengal: The 'Sari' and the Bengali 'Nari': A Dress Code." *Gender and Modernity*, edited by Amitava Chatterjee, Setu Prakashani, 2015, pp. 273-92.

Wolf, Naomi. *The Beauty Myth: How Images of Beauty Are Used against Women*. Vintage, 1991.

3.

Beautiful/Ugly

Lori Don Levan

Every day you have to get up, but it can be hard if you are feeling sick or if it is just too hard to face the day. Sometimes, there is no difference. It is often an inner voice that breaks through the confusion of life to tell you to hang on.

As an artist, I have often turned the tables on myself as I search for subject matter to explore. A time came not too long ago when I had to face my own demons or be swallowed by them.

I created a self-portrait project where over a period of five months, I took photographs of myself and documented the mundaneness of my life in an attempt to examine the state of my existence and the depression I had fallen into.

This ongoing project connects me, in various and challenging ways, to my experiences of aging, disability, mental health, and the contrasting binary of beautiful and ugly.

It is an attempt to tell my story as an aging, white, single, childless, and cisgendered woman living in a world where all of those things intersect with my fatness, which is sometimes viewed as an abomination.

What follows is a small excerpt from that project.

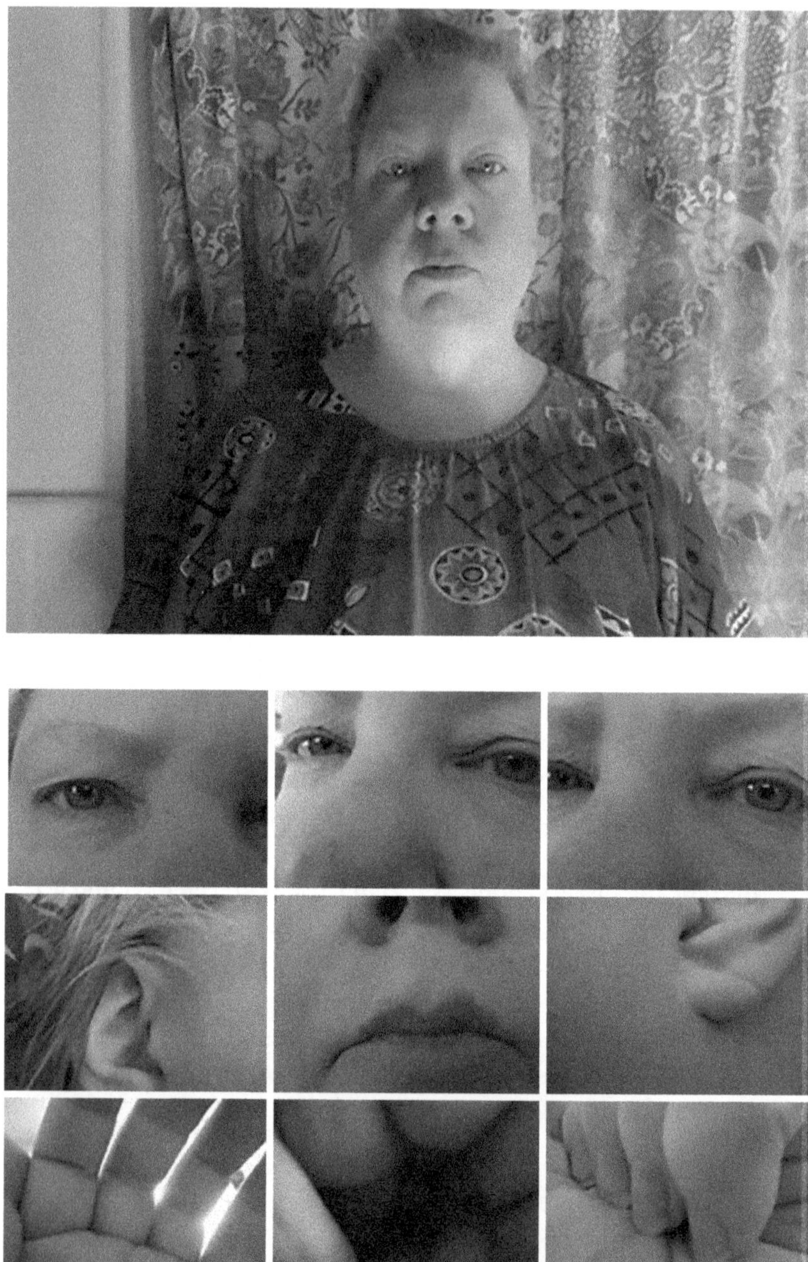

The camera can bring comfort when examining the mundane as I confront my flaws in small doses, but I am sometimes startled by the image in the mirror.

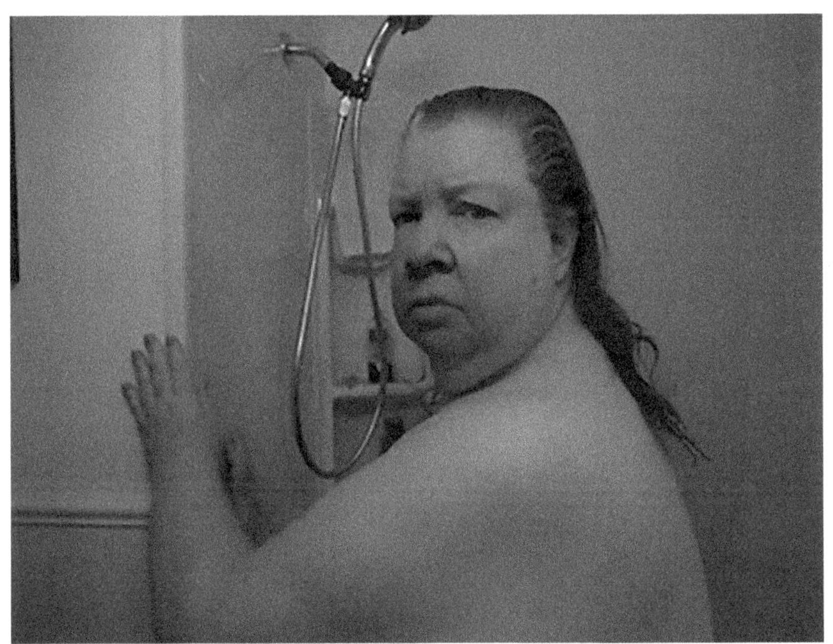

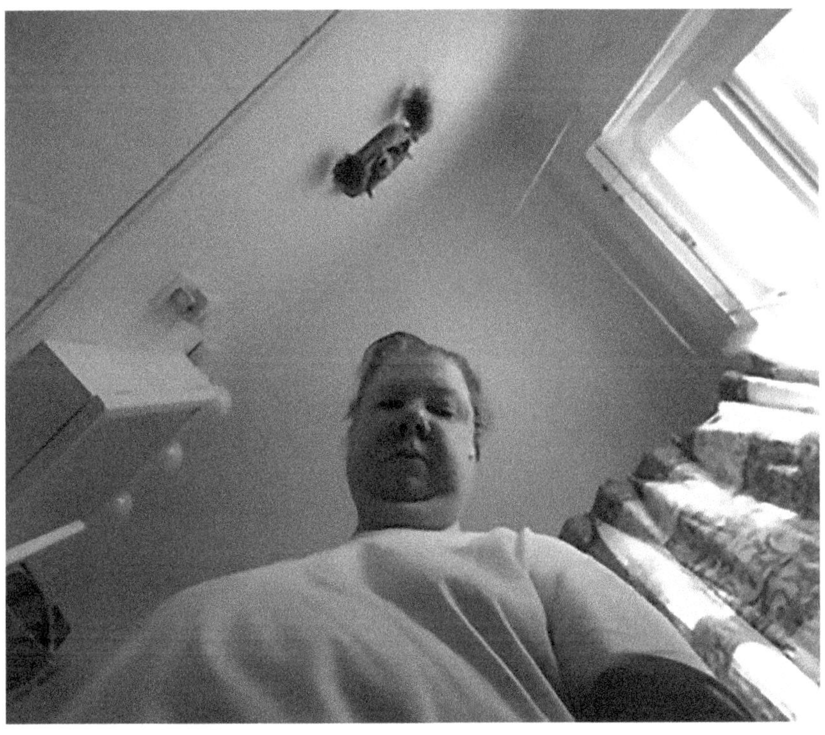

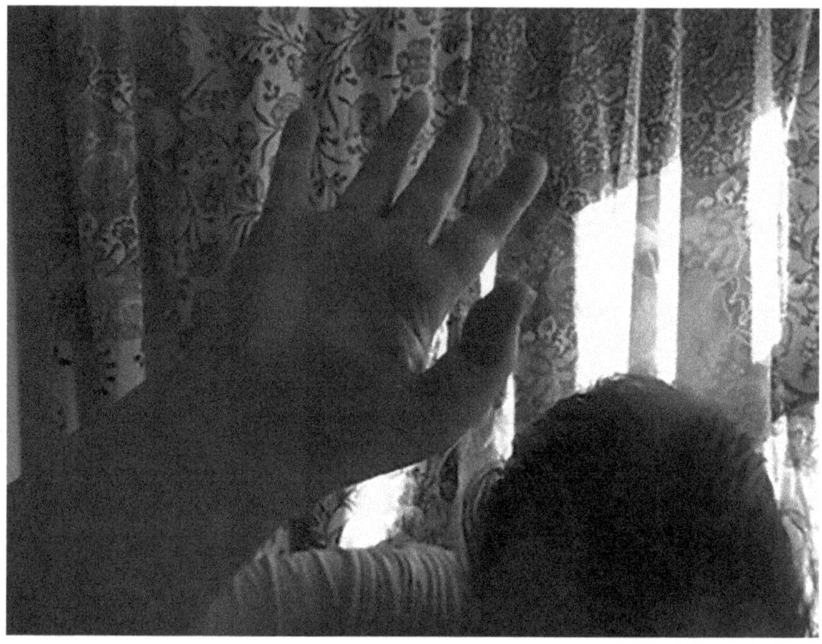

Above and below, am I looking back on myself as a child or falling into an unknown future? More questions will come as I continue to work on this project, which will hopefully guide me towards a new beginning.

4.

"I'm Not Fat. I'm Pregnant": A Critical Discussion of Current Debates in Body Size, Fatness, Pregnancy, and Motherhood

Alys Einion

Introduction

The swelling belly and rounded body shape of the childbearing woman has been negatively redefined in current medicalized discourses, which dominate the content and implementation of maternity care, particularly in Western contexts. Regardless of individual differences, race, genetics, or individual health or level of fitness, the dominant tropes of technocratic medicine continue to disempower women through the regulation of their experience of motherhood, culminating in basing of risk status (high and low risk) on body mass index (BMI), which is fundamentally flawed. In this critical, analytical, and unashamedly challenging chapter, I will utilize my feminist perspective to explode the myths of the fat reproducing body and its place within the wider lexicon of fat-shaming medicalized discourse around motherhood, which is solely focused on labelling women as deviant if they do not fit arbitrary and unfounded norms that limit their individual choices.

Women, Obesity, Negativity, Stigma, and Blame

For some women, pregnancy is the first time their body shape is viewed as acceptable. The pregnant body is supposed to bloom and to be rounded, softer, and larger. However, there is a disturbing trend towards women disliking their pregnant bodies and their increasing size because it transgresses the deeply internalized Western beliefs that to be anything other than lean and thin is wrong (Hesse-Biber et al). The literature shows that "fat women experience more prejudice and discrimination than thinner women and men of any weight in the media, the workplace, romantic relationships, and educational and health care systems" (Chrisler 608).

The obstetric literature is aligned with a negative response to fat pregnant bodies. Paternalistic and patronizing tones in the style of articles, which unashamedly condemn "the obese pregnant woman" (Gunatilake and Perlow 106), position fat mothers as villains and social criminals, who are systematically destroying the very future of the human race. Although there may be (disputed) links between maternal BMI, increased body fat, and certain risks of suboptimal pregnancy outcomes, the universal approach to obesity stigma and shaming women for their body size derives predominantly from the social construction of obesity as an irresponsible state of being. The fat pregnant woman is viewed as consuming healthcare and other state resources as avidly as she is believed to consume mountains of unhealthy food while refusing to move from her sofa. This viewpoint is associated with the cultural critique of female poverty as well as with "negative indications of personal behaviour" (Evans 439), of which obesity is the most visible and, I would argue, the most "regarded with contempt" (Evans 439).

The first role of a feminist critic is to highlight the underpinning sexist bias within healthcare services that devalues the female. Higher BMI should not be the defining factor in how women are viewed or, indeed, in the way that they are treated by healthcare providers or the state. The prevailing discourse simplifies obesity to an issue primarily founded on the "calories in, calories out" model. When health professionals produce papers that define obesity as a simple equation of indolence and overindulgence, they, unsurprisingly, reduce yet another complex biological, psychological, and social issue to an unrealistic conceptualization of behaviour, which vilifies the individual and takes no account of genetics, economics, environment, or personal history. It is well known that calorie-restricted diets not only do not work in the long term but can result in significant health problems and can actually lead to a larger body size and increased body fat. It is not news that the diet industry is founded on women failing to lose weight; it would not be so successful an industry if diets worked effectively. It is also evident that obesity cannot be used as a measure of cardiometabolic health (Tomiyama et al).

Women are constantly bombarded with messages about the desirability of food, the pleasure of chocolate, the reward of the indulgent latte after a hard day's work, the convenience of the takeaway meal. Yet one half of the population (because the diet industry and the cult of the thin is focused on women) are told that it is wrong for them to avail themselves of these social rituals and of the food being marketed to them so cleverly. Women are surrounded by an impossible paradox: the drive to be thin in order to be of value and the pressure to consume what will keep us from being thin. Being thin is equated with being healthy, but pleasure is equated with indulgence. Therefore, women receive the message that they have no right to pleasure because it will devalue them socially. It is a form of nutritional chastity: women are morally superior if they say no. I observe this all around me, in pregnant and nonpregnant friends and colleagues, all female, whose main topic of conversation is their body size or current weight-loss program. Their idea of a positive comment to one another is to suggest that someone has lost weight. That these highly skilled, highly educated, and generally very positive colleagues work in reproductive health shows just how deeply and pervasively this discourse is ingrained in our consciousness. It is indeed hard to challenge it when even a national professional association in the UK that supports, informs and insures midwives is publicly allied with a weight-loss company.

The cult of thinness is a cult whose priesthood is patriarchal and whose congregation is largely female. According to Marika Tiggeman and Amanda Pickering, women are subject to the pervasiveness of the media, which "presents women with a constant barrage of idealized images of extremely thin women, that are nearly impossible for most women to achieve" (199-200). These same authors show that only between 5 and 10 per cent of American women can achieve the thin ideal, and, therefore, the rest of the population spend their lives feeling like failures. This is compounded in pregnancy and parenting. Women who become mothers are held responsible for the future health, wellbeing, and body size of their children. They are subject to unchallenged discourses, which demand that they restrict their calories and increase their exercise, spending their scarce resources on extra physical exercise outside the milieu of home and work. A healthy diet may be a positive goal, albeit one which is unevenly available. Joyful movement may also contribute to positive acts of self-care. But these two factors are lost within the branding of the diet and exercise industries, which place unrealistic and unachievable expectations on all women and foster ignoring self-care and self-love in favour of ideals of thinness. This messaging is especially potent for pregnant women,[1] who, as I will discuss below, are subject to the greatest level of state-sanctioned surveillance they will ever experience once they become pregnant.

What does this mean for pregnant women? It means that not only are they subject to a judgmental medical gaze, which regulates their behaviour in pregnancy through threat and coercion, they are also often subject to the scrutiny of a female profession (midwifery), which enforces the overriding message of thin equals good and fat equals bad. If healthcare professionals' worldview is that body size is subject to automatic and unquestioned value judgments, this must affect how they view, respond to, and treat their clients. Socialization into a set of beliefs and ideals that values women's appearance over all other qualities is supported by professional education. It is hardly surprising that midwives, nurses, and doctors, who are constantly exposed to thinly veiled misogynistic rhetoric and discourse, are at risk of immediately judging fat pregnant women in a negative manner before they carry out any individualized health assessments. In one paper, for example, examining obesity in pregnancy, Roland et al. refer to obese pregnant women as "this group" and infer throughout that obesity is always associated with risk and that obese pregnant women are apparently homogenous. There is so much more to health than simply body size and weight.

Physiologically, obesity is a complex phenomenon, which is not reflected in current guidelines. The Royal College of Obstetricians and Gynaecologists (RCOG) in their Green Top guideline no. 72 use BMI as the sole measurement of obesity and do not adequately address individual differences or the fact that BMI was never intended to be used in pregnancy. Obesity is linked to genetic heritage as well as other factors (Iacobini et al, 51); naturally, people have widely differing body shapes and sizes and some are more predisposed to more body fat. Psychologically, obesity is related to the way that women are brought up, their beliefs about food, their experiences, and to such issues as emotional eating. It is strongly related to a history of dieting because diets fail, women regain weight, acquire more body fat, and so grow steadily larger. Socially and socioeconomically, obesity relates to availability of resources, to marketing, and to the food industry, which pumps so-called foods full of sugar and fat and sells such items at a lower price to a generation of people who do not necessarily have the time, knowledge, inclination, or resources to make choices, such as cooking for themselves. Women continue to bear the burden of the domestic sphere, and even when they are in relationships or marriages, they continue to perform most household duties compared to male spouses. Women go out to work, and on returning home, are then faced with another set of expectations that men are less subject to, that they will cook fresh food, eat a healthy diet, and only put into their pregnant bodies healthy, sanctioned foods within a limited range of calories to ensure they do not gain excessive weight during pregnancy. This is on top of the burden of maintaining feminine beauty practices and appearance, a direct form and expression of subordination (Jeffreys).

Pregnancy as a Time of Surveillance

Pregnancy is a time when women—who are already controlled, restricted, and scrutinized in almost every area of their lives—experience a new and unique level of surveillance. The current discourses of the pregnant body are diverse, but there is a worrying trend towards classifying the pregnant woman as a vehicle, a receptacle, or a walking womb more powerfully and more completely than ever before. It is no surprise that this is the result of centuries of patriarchal control of every possible dimension of women's lives and existence. The separation of the woman (the person) and her body (the vessel in which she carries her child) emphasizes both the need for control and regulation and the underlying concept that the body is something we should regard as distinct from the self.

Pregnant women in the United Kingdom (UK) have their BMI measured at the beginning of pregnancy in order to determine their risk status (RCOG). This then determines whether they are allowed to give birth at home, in a birth centre, or in an obstetric unit (a hospital). Recent guidelines show that women without complications should avoid giving birth in a hospital. Being fat, however, is viewed as a complication, which immediately increases the woman's risk of being subjected to increased surveillance, control, coercion, intervention, and iatrogenic complications such as induction of labour, limitations on mode of birth, and use of continuous fetal monitoring. These restrictions can negatively affect the physiology of birth (by restricting position and free movement in labour, for example) and can bring about a cascade of further interventions, all of which have significantly higher risks attached to them. There is also a trend of classifying obese people as irresponsible, since they are seen a drain on scarce healthcare resources.

The key issue here is that one limited measurement is being used to define these women as high risk, leaving them burdened with the significant impact of the whole risk discourse. Research and opinion are clear that using BMI as a health indicator is of limited value. Thirty years ago, Stanley Garn et al. argued that BMI is not "independent of stature," suggesting that normative weight measurements may actually differ depending on height and, thus, rendering the BMI measurement flawed. More recent research shows that "BMI is unable to distinguish between lean and fat mass" (Buss 264). Frank Nutall traces the history of obesity and BMI measurements and highlights how poor a measure of health or even body mass status BMI is. A meta-analysis of thirty-two studies looking at BMI measurements found that it was in fact not very reliable at measuring body fat (Okorodudu et al.). Body fat composition can differ according to race (Wang et al), gender (Buss), and age (Wells). Darren Brenner et al. in their study show that waist circumference is more strongly associated with serum lipid concentrations than BMI (1). Julia Buss states that "To better assess weight status, waist circumference should be included" and that "Dietary habits, physical inactivity, psychological wellbeing, and smoking status should be assessed to evaluate individual health risk" (264). However, waist circumference is not a reliable measurement during pregnancy. There are also increased rates of higher BMI among women from various minorities, such as Black and minority ethnic groups and lesbians (Yancey et al.). Such women may experience multiple intersections of stereotyping or discrimination, which shows that BMI is a limited tool for assessing overall health. However, it seems to have become the gold standard of maternity care and, thus, increases the risk burden pregnant women experience, stigmatizing them and their bodies at a time when their health and wellbeing should be optimized.

Obesity, Risk, and Health Promotion during Pregnancy and Birth

I have deliberately left until the latter half of this chapter what is almost always found at the beginning of every academic and research article on obesity in pregnancy: the associated risks. These data are, however, limited in their scope. There is sometimes little differentiation, for example, between the level of obesity in many of these articles, so it is not always possible to identify the degree of risk depending on the degree of obesity. The generalization of obesity (ranging from a woman with a BMI of twenty-six to a woman with a BMI of fifty or more) may serve to label women as high risk regardless of her individual body shape, fat stores, health and fitness, diet, activity and the like, as discussed above. Although the RCOG guidelines do differentiate between different grades of obesity, there is little evidence supporting this differentiation, and the guidelines acknowledge the limitations of evidence supporting some of its recommendations. For example, there is no evidence about whether CTG monitoring in labour is of any benefit, yet the guideline recommends this. There is an increased risk of stillbirth associated with obesity, as the RCOG guidelines show, but the aetiology of this is not well understood, and this simple association has not been proved to be causative. Emphasising this risk factor may increase women's fear and guilt during pregnancy.

Women who are classified as obese often have negative or dissatisfying experiences of care during pregnancy and birth. It is interesting to note how many of the articles cited in the reference list of the RCOG look at risk factors alongside the cost to healthcare services. This tendency to associate obesity with healthcare cost in itself can be seen as a fundamental social bias against obese people, associated with a discourse of blaming individuals (particularly women) who experience poverty (Evans), which directly feeds into the discourse of blame and stigma and an underlying (and discriminatory) assumption that obese people are social deviants. Women can, for example, receive inconsistent information and guidance from health professionals within maternity care (Oteng-Nim et al.).

Some research demonstrates that midwives—the primary point of contact and provider of care for all women in the UK—often do not give enough useful advice or support to women about exercise in pregnancy (Weir et al). The RCOG guidelines acknowledge that there is no clear standard of guidance on optimal weight gain during pregnancy. It seems that women are simply expected to access information via the leaflets and books signposted or distributed by their care providers, many of which give confusing and even contradictory guidance (Clarke and Gross). They are not then able to make informed decisions or manage their level of risk and, perhaps, will be more likely to adhere to the decisions of healthcare providers, thus losing their autonomy. There are increased risks with increased body size and weight, but these should be assessed based on individual health parameters and concomitant health issues rather than on one arbitrary and unfounded measure of obesity. The RCOG guidelines do reference these issues, but anecdotally, I have heard many stories of women who are of larger body size being automatically told they must give birth in a consultant-led unit when the RCOG guidelines state otherwise, or being referred for obstetric review, regardless of their BMI status or other healthy behaviours, simply because their BMI is above the normative values.

In the UK, referral for obstetric care means greater medical surveillance of what is and always has been a natural, human experience, for which the childbearing body is perfectly designed. Surveillance includes close monitoring of the amount of weight gained during pregnancy and a more medicalized approach to monitoring fetal development because the untamed fat pregnant body makes it harder to use traditional methods, such as symphysis-fundal height measurements, to monitor fetal growth. Thus, women of a larger body size are, for example, more likely to undergo more frequent scans—a technological intervention whose long-term effects remain difficult to ascertain. The literature shows that women are painfully conscious of their larger body size and that feelings of alienation and humiliation are associated with increased awareness of the medical gaze during pregnancy (Nyman et al). Given the fact that mental health and wellbeing is of increasing concern in pregnant people, and that stress has a negative effect on mental health and on physiological aspects of pregnancy and birth, it is irresponsible and harmful to subject women to the burden of a negative discourse based on erroneous assumptions.

Conclusions

The purpose of this discussion has been to discuss the ways in which fat women during pregnancy are subject to greater surveillance and judgement and how that surveillance, and the discourses of medicalization, glorify risk through generalization and depersonalization at the expense of individual health assessment and sensitive management of health needs. We should surely be focusing on optimizing health, not forcing women to worry about weight gain alone. Professionals' focus on weighing pregnant women and labelling their weight as problematic results in negative childbearing experiences, which could result in poorer outcomes for women and their children. Greater surveillance does not necessarily result in women engaging in health-enhancing behaviours and has the potential to alienate women from their healthcare providers. There is a very real need to challenge the underlying ideology of 'thinness' that brings about unconscious (and conscious) bias towards women and pregnant people.

I propose the need to base health assessments in childbearing on individual measures of wellness and to focus on empowering women to love, honour, and celebrate their childbearing bodies, which would overturn the risk discourse in favour of woman-centred and person-centred language and practices that directly oppose the institutionalized misogyny of the medical paradigm in childbirth. We can directly link the pervasiveness of women's discomfort and dissatisfaction with their bodies as vessels for pregnancy with the all-encompassing, socio-politically sanctioned, and utterly false obsession with unrealistic ideals of female size and shape, which are predicated on fashion, not science. This approach requires a redefinition of the very concepts that define how women see themselves, which means, for example, challenging women to see themselves as whole and complete beings rather than seeing their bodies as distinct from their minds, souls, and personalities. Once the pregnant body is viewed as the self and not as separate vessel, it may be harder for such dominant discourses of self-abnegation to take root, but this would require a radical reconceptualization of the very nature of womanhood. As Sharlene Hesse-Biber et al. (219) state: "Re-visioning femininity is not easy for women because some may be unwilling to give up the hard-earned social and economic awards they have gained by following the societal message of ultra-thinness.... Social action on the part of women to determine their own identities is an important way to challenge patriarchy's message that to strive for the thin ideal is to be empowered."

Fat pregnant women should not lose the joy and wonder of the experience of pregnancy in their worry about their body size and pregnancy outcomes. Care providers should advocate for fat-friendly maternity care while taking every opportunity to challenge the misogynistic preconceptions of fat women that continue to oversimplify a complex problem and to challenge the negative, medicalised language, which is used to alienate women from themselves and to relegate them to the status of walking womb carrying the burden of responsibility for the future of the human race. The literature shows that professionals need to be truly nonjudgmental (Knight-Agarwal et al). How they can develop a truly woman-positive approach to the bodies of their clients, when they themselves are subject to the same negative social codes and prejudices, has yet to be established.

Until such time as women no longer have to fight for the fundamental human right of control over themselves and what happens to them, especially during pregnancy, then those of us working in maternity care must carry that challenge forwards by being advocates for equality, equity, justice, and nonjudgemental practice. All healthcare professionals, but particularly midwives, should address any internalized preconceptions, stereotypes, and prejudices they may hold and consider the impact of negative social stereotypes on the health and wellbeing of women and children in both the short and long term. It is not tolerable or equitable for fat to be a generally acceptable form of social prejudice. Instead, we should share our positive awareness of pregnant women's changing physicality, honour their body shape, celebrate their ability to bear children, and value the work they engage in to be healthy and to be good, strong, and loving mothers.

Endnotes

1. Here I specifically refer to pregnant women because of the gendered nature of cultural messages and social forces relating to the child-bearing body and to female body size and appearance, which is the focus of this analysis. Usually, I would also use the term "pregnant person" to include those of other genders who are pregnant or birthing.

Works Cited

Brenner, Darren R., et al. "Comparison of Body Mass Index and Wait Circumference as Predictors of Cardiometabolic Health in a Population of Young Canadian Adults." *Diabetology & Metabolic Syndrome.* vol 2. no. 28 (2010), dmsjournal.biomedcentral.com/articles/10.1186/1758-5996-2-28. Accessed 16 Oct. 2020.

Buss, Julia. "Limitations of Body Mass Index to Assess Body Fat." *Workplace Health and Safety,* vol. 62, no. 6, 2014, p. 264.

Chrisler, Joan C. "'Why Can't You Control Yourself?' Fat *Should Be* a Feminist Issue." *Sex Roles,* vol. 66, 2012, pp. 608-26.

Clarke, P.E., and H. Gross. "Women's Behaviour, Beliefs and Information Sources about Physical Exercise in Pregnancy." *Midwifery,* vol. 20, 2004, pp. 133-41.

Devlieger, Roland, et al. "Maternal obesity in Europe: Where Do We Stand and How to Move Forward? A Scientific Paper Commissioned by the European Board & College of Obstetrics and Gynaecology (EBCOG)" *European Journal of Obstetrics and Gynecology and Reproductive Biology* vol. 201, 2016, pp. 203-208.

Evans M. "Women and the Politics of Austerity: New Forms of Respectability." *British Politics,* vol. 11, no. 4, 2016, pp. 438-51.

Furber, Christine, and Linda McGowan. "A Qualitative Study of the Experiences of Women Who Are Obese and Pregnant in the UK." *Midwifery,* vol. 27, no. 4, 2011, pp. 437-44.

Garn, Stanley, et al. "Three Limitations of the Body Mass Index." *American Journal of Clinical Nutrition,* vol. 44, 1986, pp. 996-97.

Gunatilake, Ravida, and Jordan H. Perlow. "Obesity and Pregnancy: Clinical Management of the Obese Gravida." *American Journal of Obstetrics and Gynaecology,* vol. 204, no. 2, 2011, pp. 106-19.

Heslehurst, N., et al. "Implementation of Pregnancy Weight Management and Obesity Guidelines: A Meta-Synthesis of Healthcare Professionals' Barriers and Facilitators Using the Theoretical Domains Framework." *Obesity Reviews,* vol. 15, no. 6, 2014, pp. 462-86.

Hesse-Biber, Sharlene, et al. "The Mass Marketing of Disordered Eating and Eating Disorders: The Social Psychology of Women, Thinness and Culture." *Women's Studies International Forum,* vol. 29, 2006, pp. 208-24.

Iacobini, Carla et al. 'Metabolically healthy versus metabolically unhealthy obesity.' *Metabolism* 92, pp. 51-60.

Jeffreys, Sheila. *Beauty and Misogyny: Harmful Cultural Practices in the West*. Routledge, 2005.

Knight-Agarwal, R.C., et al. 'The perspectives of obese women receiving antenatal care: a qualitative study of women's experiences.' *Women and Birth* 29:2 (2016): 189-195.

Nutall Frank Q. 'Body Mass Index: Obesity, BMI and Health: A Critical Review.' *Nutrition Today*, vol. 50, no. 3, 2015, pp. 117-128

Nyman Viola MK, et al. "Obese Women's Encounters with Midwives and Physicians during Pregnancy and Childbirth." *Midwifery*, vol. 26, no. 4, 2010, pp. 424-29.

Okorodudu, D.O., et al. "Diagnostic Performance of Body Mass Index to Identify Obesity as Defined by Adiposity: A Systematic Review and Meta-Analysis." *International Journal of Obesity*, vol. 34, 2010, pp. 791-99.

Royal College of Obstetricians and Gynaecologists. *Care of Women with obesity in Pregnancy. Green Top Guideline No. 72*, www.rcog.org.uk/en/guidelines-research-services/guidelines/gtg72/ Accessed 4 Oct. 2020.

Tiggeman, Marika, and Amanda S Pickering. "Role of Television in Adolescent Women's Body Dissatisfaction and Drive for Thinness." *International Journal of Eating Disorders*, vol. 20, no. 2, 1996, pp. 199-203.

Tomiyama, A.J., et al. "Misclassification of Cardiometabolic Health When Using Body Mass Index Categories in NHANES 2005-2012." *International Journal of Obesity*, vol. 40, no. 5, 2016, pp. 883-86.

Wang, J., et al. "Asians Have Lower Body Mass Index (BMI) but Higher Percent Body Fat Than Do Whites: Comparisons of Anthropometric Measurements." *American Journal of Clinical Nutrition*, vol. 60, 1994, pp. 23-28.

Weir, Z., et al. "Physical Activity in Pregnancy: A Qualitative Study of the Beliefs of overweight and obese pregnant women." *BMC Pregnancy and Childbirth* 10 (2010): 18.

Yancey, Antoinette. "Obesity at the Crossroads: Feminist and Public Health Perspectives." *Signs: Journal of Women in Culture and Society*, vol. 31, no. 2, 2006, pp. 425-43.

5.

Eating While Fat: Mapping the Journey

Sam Abel and Crystal Kotow

Food is never just about nutrition. As Jennifer Brady, Jacqui Gingras, and Elaine Power assert, food carries multiple levels of emotional, social, cultural, and political meanings, which are intertwined with taste, memory, tradition, and ritual. Whether feeding themselves or others, women have complicated relationships with food, foodwork, and the body. As fat women, our relationships with eating cannot be separated from the cultural assumptions, stereotypes, drives, and fears that Susan Bordo describes as inscribed on our bodies.

This chapter will explore how visual methodologies may extend our thinking when conceptualizing complex relationships to food and will detail our experience with the body mapping process. Given the complexity of our relationships with food, we decided that the best way to explore these issues was through the visual methodology of body mapping, which is a storytelling research method focused on "life-sized human body images ... created using drawing, painting or other art-based techniques to visually represent aspects of people's lives, their bodies, and the world they live in" (Gastaldo et al. 5). Body mapping has been used to uncover experiences of HIV/AIDS, migration, chronic pain, child abuse, and a variety of other social issues. Although our body maps are deeply personal to us, we believe that they will feel intimately familiar to many women in Western society.

Why Visual Methodologies?

Sandra Weber claims that the arts provide access to qualities of life that literal language is often unable to engage. Artistic forms of research and representation can be used to generate an "improved understanding of the human condition" (Eisner 6). Elliot Eisner highlights that art in research aims to be evocative rather than solely descriptive. The evocative elements that generate emotion and imagination allow viewers to participate vicariously in the situation. Body maps, due to their size and story, allow contentious issues to be disseminated in ways that evoke empathy and understanding rather than ridicule or pathologization. We feel that body maps align with the goal of arts-based research to "unveil oppression and transform unjust social practices" by connecting with the everyday lives of real people (Finley 9).

Body mapping is a methodology that takes an asset-based approach to research (Gastaldo et. al 8). Participants are seen in a positive way, as people who have a contribution to offer social and health sciences. It recognizes participants as having expertise, experiences, and perceptions about embodiment. The method advocated by Denise Gastaldo et al. involves three components. The process first begins by outlining participants' bodies on paper so that they can work with a life-sized picture of themselves. The second component is creating a body map key that describes each element of the map in first person, which ensures that viewers are granted access to the visual narrative (Gastaldo et. al 17). Finally, after the map is created, the participant will write a brief, first-person narrative that provides a broad description about the person's life and gives context to the map and the key. Body mapping is a flexible method of knowledge creation. Although Gastaldo et al. set guidelines for where to place different elements of the body map (e.g., items related to heritage are generally placed in the bottom left corner of the map), we chose to approach each of our body maps in ways that aligned with how we wanted to tell our stories. The body map uses multiple art supplies and often has the appearance of more of a collage. Lynn Butler-Kisber describes the potential of a collage as being able to mediate understanding in new and interesting ways for both the creator and the viewer because of its "partial, embodied, multivocal, and nonlinear representational potential" (5).

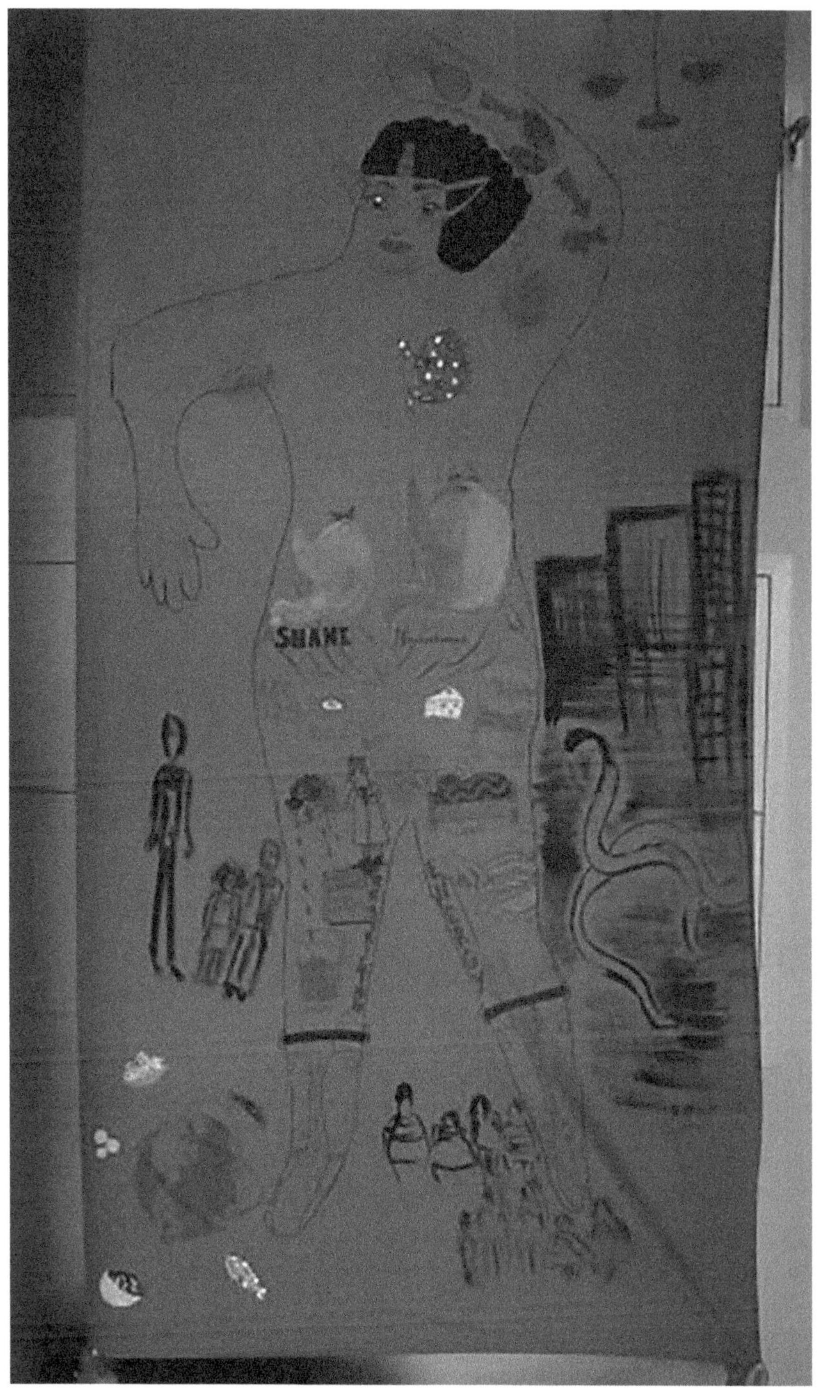

Samantha Abel's Body Map.

Artist Statement: Samantha Abel

The written word can evoke a lot, but when you read about social issues, you still maintain a distance. Seeing a visual representation of the sometimes-devastating and always life-changing impacts of social issues is visceral and eye opening.

After my body outline was traced, I began in the bottom left corner, where I considered how to demonstrate my roots and histories as they relate to food. The globe with lots of arrows represents my family's migration patterns and that I have both lived and travelled all over the world. These migration patterns have had an influence on the way my families and I cook and relate to food. Recipes change and are adapted when you live somewhere and can't get the ingredients you need or when you are trying to assimilate into a culture.

I chose the five foods represented in this corner deliberately. The matzah balls and the bowl of chana masala represent both sides of my family and their ethnic and cultural heritages. As a biracial, interfaith person, food is one thing that demonstrates the differences between my families.

My food preferences have also been influenced by the physical locations in which I have lived. The fish is a tsipoúra, native to the Mediterranean Sea. It was a frequent part of my diet when I lived in Cyprus. My mother and I would often walk down to the beach to a specific restaurant we loved, where tsipoúra was caught and served fresh daily. We would share a whole tsipoúra and a side of tabbouleh between us. The memory of these meals is tied up in my nostalgia for Cyprus and my childhood.

My body has three stomachs, including one where my heart would be. My first stomach is emotional, because I am an emotional eater and I have been taught to be ashamed of this. My second stomach is linked to dieting and medical shaming. My final stomach represents things that nourish me.

My right arm shows my journey from someone who eats meat, to being vegetarian, to eating fish again. This arm represents the struggle between taking an ethical stance about food and listening to the messages and signals my body sends me.

Part of the body mapping process is to show marks on or under your skin. I immediately represented my stretch marks accurately because food has fuelled my body to grow and change in ways that have left their marks. I also chose to show my leg braces and the marks they have caused as well as the pain. My disability affects my ability to be nourished when I am in pain and do not have the energy to cook.

The top right corner is supposed to demonstrate your goals and what you are striving towards. I chose to draw a scale to represent balance. Balance with food is a very hard thing for me. I feel like I am always striving to achieve balance, but various things get in the way. Since being in graduate school, my nutritional balance has been destroyed. I feel like the ever-changing schedules and never-ending workdays of academia make nourishment extremely difficult.

Overall, creating a body map was a more difficult process than I had anticipated. The emotional aspects of creating the map were more overwhelming than I was expecting. Although I don't usually get hung up on the "correct" way to do things, especially when they are artistic, I did feel some trepidation about doing things "wrong". I ultimately skipped several of the steps that weren't working for me or didn't feel right; I embraced my artistic style and produced a piece of art/research that I feel very happy with and proud of.

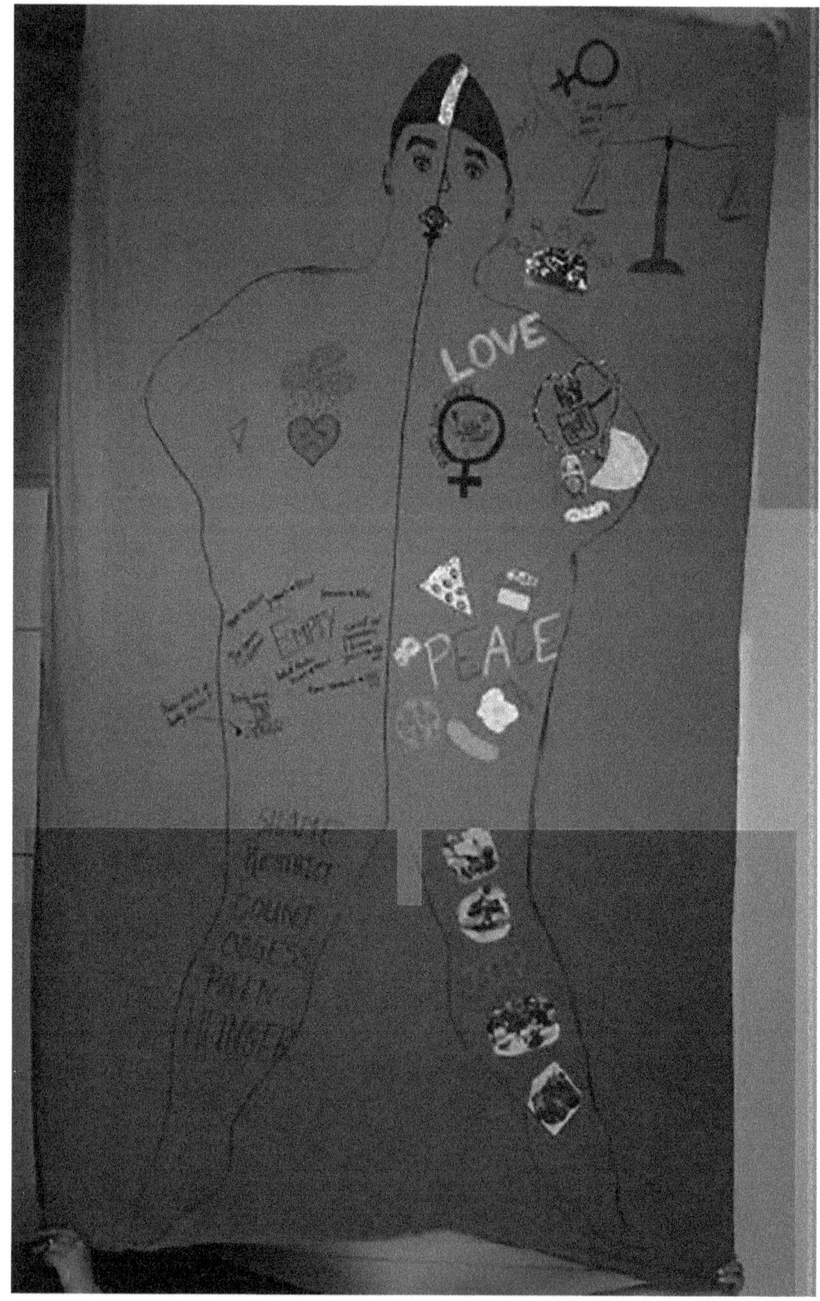

Crystal Kotow's Body Map.

Artist Statement: Crystal Kotow

My food journey has been significantly influenced by the diet and weight-loss industries as well as by family, friends, feminism, and the fat acceptance movement. My body map tells these stories.

This map reads as a journey—an ongoing journey. One side of the map represents my relationship with food during my early twenties when I engaged in severely disordered eating and exercise patterns that resulted in significant weight loss (approximately one hundred pounds in five months). Interestingly, even though my body shrunk down to a size eighteen—still fat by societal standards—I hated myself more than ever. Symbolic of this time in my life, two focal points on this side of the map include a list of foods and their calorie counts surrounding the word "empty" on my stomach as well as a series of words written down my leg representing emotions and actions that ruled my life. I was killing myself but believed I was living a healthy and sustainable lifestyle. And, of course, at every turn there was a friend or family member validating my shrinking body and all the hard work I was doing.

I wrote "How does a body thrive?" just outside my stomach. This is a serious question. Quite literally, how does a body thrive on calorie deficits? Additionally, how does a body thrive when, not just physical, but emotional violence is being enacted upon it? It was a constant struggle. I struggled with never feeling sated. I struggled with food obsession as a result of constant hunger. I struggled with the idea that nothing about me was good enough, even though I was consistently shrinking my body to fit ideals I was told needed to be met. And when my body had finally had enough of being starved and started gaining back the lost weight, I struggled with body image and food relationships for the next five years until my weight stabilized.

When I was twenty-five and working on my master's research about media representations of fat women, my life changed drastically upon discovering fat activism. The other half of the body map tells the story of my complex relationship with food now.

Feminism and fat activism symbols and phrases represent how I currently live my life. I speak my politics at every opportunity, and they determine who I love, what I love, and the way I love. Nothing about me is gentle or subtle. My body takes up space, and my politics are radical. I quote the lyrics "I have always been a storm," which is a metaphor for the way my politics often destroy people's preconceived notions of me and of social issues I openly discuss. Sometimes relationships are damaged as well. Not to be overlooked is the fact that many storms move through an area, leaving it refreshed and revitalized, something I hope I do for others when I vocalize my politics—especially around food and diet culture.

The remainder of this half of the map showcases a joyful relationship with food, symbolizing my love of cooking for others and of food-related family traditions. I also point to my close relationship with my mother, which has been forged by our mutual love of caring for others and ourselves through food.

I'd be remiss if I didn't acknowledge that despite my relationship with food shifting in a more positive direction, I still struggle with food issues. I use food to manage stress, an effect I experience in scores as a graduate student. Healing my relationship with food was one of the most revolutionary things I've done for my physical, mental, and emotional health; however, the journey is ongoing, sometimes circular, and will always be challenging.

Conclusion

Although eating could be defined simply as a process that we participate in to survive, how we relate to food goes far beyond survival. Food and eating are tied up in nourishment, journey, balance, and a host of other ideas, places, cultures, and histories.

Our relationships with food are always complex. How we approach food and eating is further complicated by fatness. Body mapping provides an appropriate methodology to explore these complexities because it is understood to be a relational, knowledge-disseminating, capacity-building, and action-mobilizing tool. Creating body maps with people who have experienced similar struggles is a powerful and transformative experience. Our process made the relational and social benefits of body mapping very clear to us. It felt important to be working with someone who was also creating a body map, as opposed to self-administering or working with a therapist. We both required each other's support and probably would not have continued had we been mapping alone. There is a lot of trust required when body mapping with someone, and we emerged from the exercise closer than we were before.

In the summer of 2015, we piloted a body mapping workshop at a conference specifically focused on fatness. We were initially concerned that the process might be too personal for people to want to participate, but we had so many participants sign up that we had to turn people away.

We found that the transformative space that we had created when together also translated to a larger group, and that it felt powerful to explore fatness visually in a shared space. As fat activists and scholars, we are excited to continue to look for ways that body mapping can be incorporated into ours and others' work.

Works Cited

Bordo, Susan. *Unbearable Weight: Feminism, Western Culture, and the Body*. Oakland, CA: University of California Press, 2003.

Brady, Jennifer, Jacqui Gingras, and Elaine Power. "Still Hungry: A Feminist Perspective on Food, Foodwork, the Body, and Food Studies." *Critical Perspectives in Food Studies*, edited by Anthony Winson, Jennifer Sumner, and Mustafa Koç, Oxford University Press, 2012, pp. 122-35.

Butler-Kisber, Lynn. "Collage as Inquiry." *Handbook of the Arts in Qualitative Research: Perspectives, Methodologies, Examples, and Issues*, edited by J. Gary Knowles and Ardra L. Cole, Sage, 2008, pp. 265-76.

Eisner, Elliot. "Art and Knowledge." *Handbook of the Arts in Qualitative Research: Perspectives, Methodologies, Examples, and Issues*, edited by J. Gary Knowles and Ardra L. Cole, Sage, 2008, pp. 3-12.

Finley, Susan. "Arts-Based Research." *Handbook of the Arts in Qualitative Research: Perspectives, Methodologies, Examples, and Issues*, edited by J. Gary Knowles and Ardra L. Cole, Sage, 2008, pp. 72-83.

Gastaldo, Denise, et al. *Body-Map Storytelling as Research: Methodological Considerations for Telling the Stories of Undocumented Workers through Body Mapping*. University of Toronto, 2012, http://www.migrationhealth.ca/sites/default/files/Bodymap_storytelling_as_reseach_HQ.pdf. Accessed 10 March 2015.

Weber, Sandra. "Visual Images in Research." *Handbook of the Arts in Qualitative Research: Perspectives, Methodologies, Examples, and Issues*, edited by J. Gary Knowles and Ardra L. Cole, Sage, 2008, pp. 42-55.

6.

(Not) Too Fat to Tango

LC Di Marco

Left
Right
Forward
Turn
Back
Repeat
Flop
Roll
Drop
On the floor
Close the door
No more…snore
Right to laugh ~
Be happy
Prized to live ~
Passion
Get up off that floor ~
Dance, Smile, Laugh

Party starts when the fat lady sings
Grab a friend to the floor and dance
Let's do the tango
Time to revitalize
The heart
The beauty
The I AM ~~~~~~~~~~~~~~~

7.

"Who's Afraid of the Big Fat Feminist": An Autoethnographic Account of Fatness in Academic Feminist Spaces

Melanie Stone and Allison Taylor

This is an autoethnographic[1] account of our experiences as self-identified fat, feminist graduate students in a women's studies graduate program. By discussing our experiences in an interview, we use autoethnography to speak to the impact of the university institution on our negotiations of academic feminist spaces. We draw upon our embodied experiences of fatness to challenge the harmful, exclusionary, and ideologically laden discourse of the "desirable" feminist.

*

Melanie: How do you experience and negotiate academic spaces, such as classrooms, as a fat, feminist graduate student?

Allison: The first thing that pops into mind is the issue of fitting. When I walk into a classroom, the first thing I look at is whether the seats are going to fit [my body]. As a student not fit[ing] sends a message maybe that your body isn't intended to be there. But especially as a teaching assistant (TA), the first feeling you have is embarrassment because you're flowing out of the seat. When your students look to you, I feel like they're supposed to see you as an authority figure, and if you're sitting uncomfortably, sweating, squirming, that's not the picture of authority that is often conveyed. I also think, for example, of walking down aisles during an exam as my hips don't necessarily fit nice and neatly and I'm brushing off people's papers.[2]

Melanie: I would say the same thing. There's something strange about being a fat feminist [graduate] student who is supposed to exist in a feminist environment and always having to speak up and say, "Hey. can we get a classroom where the chairs aren't eleven inches wide?" We're always squished on top of our students. I look at a lot of issues of accessibility, and I think classrooms aren't accessible to many bodies. Even in a women's studies program, I still worry a lot about my image as a TA and how my clothes fit and how I'm being portrayed at the front of the room and what my students are seeing. I wonder, are they thinking "No wonder she's interested in feminism and body image" when I talk about health. I'm always nervous about how my students are interpreting my appearance. I spend a lot of time the first couple classes, dressing in a particular way to "flatter" my body, but by the end [of the term], that goes out the window, but, yes, I always worry about what image I'm projecting, for new women's studies students and whether they are taking me seriously as a fat feminist.[3]

Allison: Even the topics that are covered in classrooms oftentimes [are exclusionary of fatness]. Fatness is never front and centre. Maybe it is in a few courses that are specifically centered on bodies, but even there, it's maybe one week. Even then, so much of the time is spent [simply] unpacking the problematic conceptions that people have about fat bodies.

Melanie: Yeah, I think also just the way that we've started to make women's studies less about advocacy and more about being safe and palatable or something.... I've been in a few [women's studies] classes where the professor has been outright fatphobic. Saying things like "I'm not an ugly person," "women's studies professors can be hot," [and] "we're not all feminist stereotypes." Like [it's their responsibility] to somehow please the eye to be taken seriously by new students. And that is still upheld in some feminist spaces.... I worry about this sort of obsession with presenting a "nice" version of feminism and that's where a lot of discussions [of fatness become] peripheral to that message ... but if we're not sort of centring the experiences of [fat bodies] or if we're not making our classrooms accessible, what are we doing as feminists and what is that going to look like?

Melanie: So how have you encountered fat shaming or fatphobia in academic spaces, as either a TA or a graduate student?

Allison: The first instance that comes to mind is having a professor read over my work, which is on queer fat femmes, and ask, "Who is this important for? I don't understand." I think that [such an] immediate dismissal of my work [often occurs] because [many people, including fellow scholars, don't have] that critical fat studies lens. [They perceive] what we're talking about as endorsing fatness, [which they] write off as unhealthy or bad. That [might] stem from the larger issue of people just simply not being aware of fat studies or [the way our society so openly allows for people] being fatphobic.

Melanie: I've seen similar things in and around departments, too. For example, advertising for women's studies courses never includes fat bodies, and I'm always surprised by this because we're here, and this is important. There's a picture in [our department, advertising a course about pregnancy and fertility], and there's these two tiny, white[4] bellies, without a stretch mark, without any fat present. There's no body hair that we can see, and I don't know about you, but that doesn't represent my body, and it certainly didn't represent my body when I was pregnant, and it bothers me every time I see it. I wonder why we're scared to advertise for our courses in this way, without sort of encouraging looks of fatness, even when looking at pregnant women. [Some of our advertising has] great images, but when I was scanning them the other day, and this is a lot of posters, there just aren't any fat bodies. And I don't know if we've done it subconsciously, or if those images just aren't readily available, or if we are trying to pander to this, safe, kind, "pretty" version of feminism that will just get bums in seats. But whose bums? That's concerning to me. So I've had that issue, and definitely the same thing with the shape of chairs, and [spaces or seating arrangements] that have just been difficult to get into and out of. And when I go to meetings, even for our union, oftentimes I have to tell them that this isn't an accessible space and then it's like you're making a lot of noise but ... there is definitely not much commitment to accessibility or fat accommodation even within student advocacy groups or feminist spaces. That is frustrating and infuriating.

Allison: [Accessibility is important, too, for] navigating [general] spaces on campus. I remember sitting in a student lounge once, and a woman ... very directly walks over to me and hands me a pamphlet about her weight loss centre and says "You're welcome" and then walks away. She didn't hand it out to anyone else because I was the only fat person in the room. So even that idea of feeling so visible and so vulnerable in campus spaces [ties in here]. If even our feminist posters won't [portray] fat bodies and if there's no representation [of fat bodies] then what kind of message does this send about who belongs here, who doesn't, what kind of bodies we're accepting, who we're not.

Melanie: I know certainly I wouldn't feel comfortable doing a lot of social events or things after hours because the promotion for these things and who's included at these places is usually smaller students so yeah, absolutely. That takes us into the next question: Do you think that program promotion and sustainability of women's studies programs has had an impact on the continued marginalization of fat bodies?

Allison: Yes! Representation and visibility are so important, especially for fat bodies. [Fatness] is very much a material identity and experience, and if you're not seeing representations of yourself, I think that automatically sends a message by way of exclusion. I also think that you [touch on something very important] when you talk about women's studies [and/or feminism] being made palatable. [There is a] sort of mainstream, or arguably verging on postfeminist, discourse of "I'm not a lesbian. I'm not ugly. I'm [not] fat. I'm a hot feminist! I'm a fun feminist! You can make a sexist joke, [and] I'm going to laugh because we know that's not really how it is now." But for a lot of folks [sexism, homophobia, racism, and fatphobia] are [still very real sites of oppression], and I think it is especially for fat [folks]. Such rhetoric only further entrenches that sexism, homophobia, racism, and fatphobia, as well as other oppressions.

Melanie: I think we're now so focused on bums in seats to keep sustaining funding that we're not going to project that image of the awesome fat femme professor [for example]. We're not going to do that because we think that there's something unsafe about her, and [although] we may not explicitly say that, we'll just erase her from any brochures or any promotional materials. She's not a safe representation of our program. She doesn't model the "good non-threatening pretty feminist" that will make women's studies programs appeal to the masses. We've watered it down a bit to make it easier for fatphobia to exist, but I think in doing that we've created a toxic situation and environment for people, you know, who are experiencing fatphobia and allowing people to be fatphobic in our spaces with institutional support.

Allison: It's also not uncommon to overhear in feminist spaces talk of "I just want to lose five pounds" or "I've started this diet" or "My pair of jeans that didn't fit for the longest time finally do. I've managed to do it; my [weight loss] goal is met." There's so much talk of bodies and of weight loss and of fatness in such problematic ways. I'm not suggesting that people [should] police themselves, but I think there's a real lack of awareness of... well what does this mean when you're saying this sort of thing to a fat woman? I'm not going to sit there and congratulate you because you're telling me how excited you are to not look like me. I think that this [putting down and marginalization of fat bodies] happens all too often in feminist spaces, in women's studies departments, [and] maybe that [comes] down to the fact that fatness just isn't taken seriously as an axis of oppression.

Melanie: That's very true. What do you think the solutions are for women's studies programs given the boundaries of a neoliberal institution that is often ableist and fat shaming?

Allison: Going back to [the topic of] visibility, I would like to see inclusive promotional materials. I would also like to see fatness talked about in a more substantive way in classrooms—talk that isn't simply "dispelling fat myths 101" and talking about the BMI [body mass index] or health. Instead, I would like to see [us take these discussions further] and attention be [paid] to what [the] marginalization of fat bodies looks like, or rad fatties, who might even be "bad" fatties,[5] because why do discussions about fatness even need to be linked to health? I think that [idea] in itself perpetuates these [healthist, fatphobic] messages implicitly in a way. Substantive engagements with fatness in our classrooms are important.

Melanie: I agree. I think visibility is key and that means that when we're looking to hire people [as] faculty, we take seriously this engagement with fat studies and perhaps bring different bodies and different people to the table ... that's needed all over. I think for me it's [also] an accessibility issue. Our schools are just inaccessible, so I would just like to see us, especially as a women's studies faculty, and in women's studies spaces, choose classrooms that aren't fat shaming and aren't exclusionary to people who are bringing mobility aids or assistive animals or assistive devices of any kind. I would just like to see accessibility improved across campus and that would improve access for all students. I would also like to ... ensure that we are not making fatphobic comments in our lectures and we have to encourage discussion about fatness in these spaces. And then, finally, I'd really like to see us stop apologizing for what we look like and who we are as academics to these students who have the wrong idea of what feminism is. It seems we spend a lot of time reassuring them that feminists aren't scary. I don't understand this. Why can't we be frightening? Why can't our bodies and our voices challenge them? Why can't we take up space? Why do we owe students new to feminism a watered down and contained version of feminism? We aren't helping them get the right idea when we say "We're not THAT kind of feminist. Obviously feminists can also be super hot and super skinny," as you said. I think it just goes back to not buying that feminism needs to look a certain way to undergraduate students in order to be important. I want them to know that you are just as valuable and respected as a fat feminist as you are as a thin one and that they don't owe anyone containment and "safe " bodies. That you can exist in many ways.

Allison: Don't apologize for your size! After all, who says feminism can't be flab-ulous?

Endnotes

1. Autoethnography is a methodology in which the researcher draws on personal experience to explore and better understand broader social and cultural phenomena.
2. This makes me think of Rosemarie Garland-Thomson's theory of misfitting. By emphasizing the relationality of mis/fitting and asserting that there is no problem inherent to the body that does not fit, her misfit theory removes blame from individual bodies (Garland Thomson 597). Therefore, when analyzing why we, as fat women, misfit, the answer does not lie with our bodies. Rather, the problem inheres in the juxtaposition between our bodies and aca-

demic environments. The problem is a neoliberal institution that marginalizes fat bodies.

3. I have frequently had conversations with other fat students and with disabled students about the way their bodies are allowed to move in spaces. For example, if you are a professor or TA and expected to facilitate an exam but your body cannot move through the aisles or stairs and spaces with ease, because of inaccessible space, do students perceive these limitations as your own? Do they attribute the deficits of the organization as deficits in the individual? Do they consider you professional when they see you struggle in a space which is not designed for you? We must call upon feminist and disability studies programs to evaluate classroom set ups and ask who is and is not welcome there.
4. It would be an oversight to not at least mention race in our discussion of fat, academic feminisms. Race is not centered in our interview, and this is a limitation of our contribution to this discussion. We would, however, like to recognize that an overarching flaw in fat studies tends to be the marginalization of analyses that include race. Accordingly, we urge scholars to analyze the role of race in future discussions of fat, academic feminisms.
5. For discussion of the "rad" and "bad" fattie, see V. Chalklin.

Works Cited

Chalklin, V. "Obstinate Fatties: Fat Activism, Queer Negativity, and the Celebration of 'Obesity." *Subjectivity,* vol. 9, 2016, pp. 107-125.

Garland-Thomson, Rosemarie. "Misfits: A Feminist Materialist Disability Concept." *Hypatia,* vol. 26, no. 3, 2011, pp. 591-609.

8.

The Rock Goddess in Large

Beatrice Hogg

All I wanted was a new tee shirt. I have a lot of tee shirts, but most of my tees are of the unisex variety. In August 2007, I tried to buy a girly tee in Las Vegas.

For most of my life, I refused to wear a tight-fitting girly tee. Being a large-bosomed African American woman was rarely a blessing. I still remember the employee picnic in the mid-eighties when my inebriated supervisor took me aside and whispered, "For a small woman, you sure have a large chest." After I accented a low-cut white dress with body glitter at an office Christmas party, the next day some men in the office left a plastic pig on my desk, with its teats covered with silver sparkles. Wearing something form fitting left me open for ridicule or unwelcomed sexual advances. I wore big tops and tee shirts for the next thirty years, but when I turned fifty, I decided that I was tired of hiding behind layers of fabric. So, in the summer of my fiftieth year, I decided to get a girly tee in Vegas.

Lots of people go to Las Vegas for the gambling or the shows. I go for the shopping. Seduced by the Miracle Mile Shops' funky fashions, I spied a tee that called my name. It had a graphic of a Black girl with an enormous Afro, which reminded me of my beginnings as a rocker/funketeer in the seventies. I looked through the pile for a large. I pulled out a tee with an "L" on it, but apparently, the letter stood for "little." I don't know on what planet this shirt was considered a large.

The next day, I went into the Elton John shop at Caesar's Palace. Elton wasn't in town that week, but I could still take home something from his Red Piano show. Elton was the first musician I fell madly in love with, even before I had developed my aforementioned rocker/funketeer persona. When I was fourteen, I bought an Elton tee shirt at a drugstore in a local mall, after my Elton-inspired piano lesson. With that history between us, I had to get an Elton tee. I found the perfect shirt. It was a sleeveless muscle tee, with a tattoolike graphic saying "Saturday Night's Alright for Fighting," one of my favorite Elton songs. And the tee was on sale! It was destiny. I assumed it was a male-cut shirt, since it was a muscle tee, so I grabbed a medium and went to the fitting room to try it on. I almost cut off my oxygen supply. After much struggling, I got it off, just before passing out. I tried the large, and it wasn't much better. I could barely move. The salesperson seemed amused by my struggles. "Do these run small?" I asked. "Yes," she said, very haughtily, looking at me in disgust. I knew she was finishing the sentence in her head with, "and you do not." I tried on some regular unisex concert shirts, but my heart wasn't in it. Finally, I left the store empty handed and broken hearted.

What was going on? Had I entered a skewered world where everything was a least a size smaller? Elton, let alone most of his fans, couldn't fit into one of these constricting contraptions.

Still having not learned my lesson, I went to another mall the next day. In one store, I found another cool girly tee shirt. It had a graphic of a glamour girl with black hair, wearing a pink bathing suit and pink pumps, covered in tattoos. I had to have it. I looked for a large, as there was no XL. These were European tee shirts. Apparently, they don't wear extra-large girly tees in Europe. Despite my disappointments from the last two days, I grabbed the large and took it into the dressing room. It fit, but just barely. But barely would just have to be enough because this tee was coming with me. The tattooed lady was just going to have to deal with residing on my big American tatas. I had a new girly tee shirt. My tee treasure hunt was complete, or so I thought.

The next day, as I was killing time before my flight home, I noticed some tee shirts at the entrance to a bar near my hotel. One immediately caught my eye. It was a bright red shirt with a guitar and flowers on it. Across the front, it said, "Rock Goddess." That's me! The red shirt would go perfectly with the red shoes I bought a few days earlier. But as I got closer to the counter, my heart sank once again. The folded teeny-tiny squares looked too small to be clothing. I had cloth napkins bigger than these shirts. I asked the counter guy the question I had been asking all week in Vegas, "Do those shirts run small?" He nodded, "Yeah, they run really small. Even our girls who work here have to wear mediums, and they are really tiny girls. I have asked them to get larger sizes, but they won't."

I lost it and started screaming. "Why won't they? I'm a Rock Goddess! Not all Rock Goddesses are small. They come in all shapes and sizes! Where is my shirt? Where are the shirts for us bigger girls? I'm a size fourteen with big boobs! Where is my fucking tee shirt?"

The guy just looked at me as I ranted. He shrugged his shoulders. "Sorry." I looked at the unisex tee shirts, which had a graphic of a pig on them. Was someone trying to tell me something? Was I either a Rock Goddess or a pig?

So, I went home, pissed off. All I wanted was a tee shirt, a sexy, stylish rock-and-roll shirt that proudly identified me as cool, edgy, and hip. But the fashion industry doesn't want to consider me, with my 38DDDs worthy of a girly tee shirt that is flattering. They don't want Elton, Iron Maiden, or Led Zeppelin stretched across my ample bosom. Why can't I go into any store and find clothes that reflect my inner rock star? All I wanted was a "Rock Goddess" in large dammit!

The search continues. As the years have passed, my acceptance of my buxom figure has grown. I feel comfortable in V-neck tees, accented with necklaces that enhance, not hide, my breasts. I proudly wear my rock-and roll-tees, even though I am now sixty. At every concert, I attend, I get a new rock shirt. I find nice tees in thrift stores, department stores, and even online.

When I can't find a cool girly shirt, sometimes I'll get a men's tee in medium that will hug my curves. But I still wear my large men's tees, too, when I feel like it and never to hide my body. Sometimes, men's tees are made better than the women's shirts, another frustration of mine. I have no idea how many tee shirts I have in my closet these days. I buy expensive, supportive bras that are attractive and functional, always reminding me to walk with my shoulders back and my head held aloft. A few years after that Vegas trip, I worked on a newspaper series on breast cancer. After talking to survivors, I learned to appreciate my healthy assets even more. When I feel like complaining about the price of a bra or a tee, I remember that even with a family history of cancer, I have been spared so far. If my figure in a form-fitting tee shirt causes stares, I ignore them.

In January 2017, I went to Vegas for my sixtieth birthday. The bar with the "Rock Goddess" tee shirts and the store where I bought that glamour girl shirt were long gone. On my birthday, I strolled in the Forum Shops in Caesar's Palace wearing a tight tee and a form-fitting leather jacket. I browsed in designer shops where tiny women's jackets were labeled "large." But I didn't care. I was happy, healthy, and looking good. I passed the shop with the Elton John tees, but I didn't even stop. I'll wait until Elton is in town, and I can finally realize my dream of seeing him perform. That evening, I went to a rock club with a friend, wearing a low-cut bright pink top. On that night, I realized that no matter the size of the tee or the size of my bra, I am a Rock Goddess.

(Update: I finally saw Elton in San Francisco on September 13, 2019, and, yes, I bought a damn tee shirt!)

9.

The Unpopularity of Being Fat and Black in Popular Culture: A Case Study on Gabourey Sidibe

Simone Samuels

"Pretty women are OVERRATED" (Cox, "Pretty Women"). That was the gospel according to Pastor Justin Cox, a popular speaker and founder of Justin Cox Ministries (formerly PC4 Ministries). He posted a video on YouTube in which he intimated that if a woman was spiritually earnest, seeking a relationship with God and beautiful on the inside, then it would not matter what she looked like on the outside—he would date her.

His incredulous YouTube viewers took him to task and asked if he would date the main character from the movie *Precious*—Claireece "Precious" Jones, played by African American actress Gabourey Sidibe. Interestingly, his viewers did not ask him if he would date Beyoncé or Kim Kardashian. Instead, they asked him if he would date Precious. But why Precious?

It almost goes without saying that Sidibe's character Precious is arguably the best affront to conventional attractiveness: she's fat[1] and she's Black, physical attributes that have historically been considered ugly. The character Precious is a dark-skinned, obese[2] teenager. Her very aesthetic grates against cultural norms of conventional beauty. It is interesting that when viewers wanted to think of the ugliest, most unattractive, most sexually unappealing person they could fathom, they chose someone both fat and Black. Although I suppose Pastor Justin tried to remain pastoral and give Precious the benefit of the doubt, his initial commentary worked to ironically reinforce the other viewers' comments – that Precious was undateable, no matter how "holy" you think are.[3]

Precious's appearance (fat and Black) not only plays a role in how she is perceived and treated by others but also plays a role in how she sees and treats herself. Gabourey Sidibe is also fat and Black, but the similarities stop there. Admittedly, her appearance plays a role in how she is perceived and treated by others—the media, Hollywood, fans, and the like. But unlike Precious, Sidibe's appearance thankfully does not play a role in how she sees herself.

Gabourey Sidibe has always interested me. She doesn't look like any other actor that I've seen on the big screen. Interviews showcase her bubbly character, and her movies highlight her undeniable talent. The woman can act. The prevailing theme surrounding Sidibe's existence, however, never centres around her ability. The conversation is always about her unsuitability—to suitors and to mainstream media—on account of her race and size. Hers is a different story from that of other mainstream actors. For one, despite her obvious, recognized, award-winning talent, and effervescent personality, despite her intelligence and confidence and class, despite her sweetness and her laugh and her ambition, Sidibe has been the target of incessant mockery and vitriolic trolling primarily because of her dark skin tone and weight.

Black dark-skinned women are often considered less than classically beautiful, to coin a term Alessandra Stanley used in her now infamous *New York Times* piece in describing the gorgeous actress Viola Davis (Stanley). In her piece, titled "Weighting to Be Seen: Race, Invisibility and Body Positivity," Sonya Renee Taylor astutely points out the following: "Our society tells us fatness is not beautiful. Blackness is historically not beautiful. So even while battling weight stigma and reclaiming size diversity as beautiful, the presence of Blackness complicates the narrative ... [Sidibe's] large size and dark skin make her an outsider even in movements of inclusivity"—such as the body positive movement.

Not only are Black women and fat women and—Lord help us—fat, Black women considered less attractive, they are also assumed to live a miserable existence. For example, as briefly alluded to above, Sidibe is often confused and conflated with her Precious character. At a photo shoot on lower Broadway, one woman exclaimed: "You look totally opposite to your character" to which Sidibe responded, "Thanks. I'm actually ... not her" (qtd. in Murphy). Sidibe later commented on attaining the role of Precious saying, "They try to paint the picture that I was this downtrodden, ugly girl who was unpopular in school and in life, and then I got this role and now I'm awesome. But the truth is that I've been awesome, and then I got this role" (qtd. in Murphy). As Kate Harding noted years ago, when Sidibe's stardom was on the ascent for her breakthrough role in *Precious*, she was a woman not struggling "with debilitating body-related shame and anxiety." How infuriating for those who believe fat equals misery (Williams).

Many have also wrongly assumed that Sidibe's love life mirrored that of her character's—turbulent, abusive, and/or non-existent. In fact, Sidibe has an active love life (Brown) and has been spotted at times hanging out with her boyfriend (Bossip). The director of *Precious,* Lee Daniels, once expressed, "Gabourey is unequivocally comfortable in her body, in a very bizarre way.[4] Either she's in a state of denial or she's so elevated that she's on another level. I had no doubt that she had four or five boyfriends, easily" (qtd. in Murphy). When asked if that was true, Sidibe cheekily responded by saying "It's a gross underestimate" (qtd. in Jeffries). She went on to recount a story of a tardy guy she once dated. On being made to wait, Sidibe said, "I told him don't, don't don't! I'm not a regular girl. I just got off a plane from France. You need to check yourself" (qtd. in Murphy). Assumptions about Sidibe's personal life are made based on the myth that fat, Black women are asexual, unattractive, and undesirable.

The myth carries over to the small screen as well. When Sidibe's character "Becky Williams" had a much talked about love scene with her conventionally handsome boyfriend on the TV series *Empire*, there was considerable backlash online. "It was like they were more comfortable with the rape scene in *Precious* than the love scene in *Empire*," she told BuzzFeed News (qtd. in Wieselman). Viewers who were shocked couldn't grasp that her very fat, very Black body was sexually desirable and that she actually had a boyfriend.

In response, Sidibe proudly stated, "I, a plus sized, dark-skinned woman, had a love scene on primetime television. I had the most fun ever filming that scene even though I was nervous. But I felt sexy and beautiful and I felt like I was doing a good job" (qtd. in Wieselman). Sidibe went on to express her desire to see more love scenes like hers on primetime television. But will there be more to come? There may be more love scenes on TV featuring voluptuous women, but will there be more TV and movie productions featuring Sidibe? Some say that on account of her size and colour, the answer is no.

Margot Magowan wrote a piece for the *SanFran Gate* titled "Gabourey Isn't Too Fat for Hollywood—She's Too Black." She alludes to the fact that many posit that Sidibe will have trouble finding a role in Hollywood because of her size and colour. "Sidibe," Magowan continues, "doesn't conform to Hollywood's narrow beauty requirements for romantic leads and stars: actresses should be white women, preferably blonde."

Never one to mince words, radio personality and shock jock Howard Stern once said that "The best is when they go for Best Actress ... it's Sandra Bullock, and then there's Helen Mirren and there's Meryl Streep and then you go, there's the most enormous, fat, Black, chick, Gabourey Sidibe." He also called Oprah Winfrey, "a filthy liar [for] telling an enormous woman the size of a planet that she's going to have a career" (qtd. in Hova). Of note is that in listing the other actresses mentioned—all coincidentally white, all of a conventionally acceptable body size—he does not mention their size or race at all. However, when commenting on Gabourey Sidibe, not only is she fat, she's Black.

In one breath, Stern normalizes thinness and whiteness—whiteness as normal and ubiquitous and so mundane that it need not be mentioned. More troubling is the lack of representation of fat Black women (or fat women in general, but fat women of colour in particular) in love scenes in which their weight is not the focus or not the story line. Marion Wright Edelman once wrote, "You cannot be what you cannot see." If curvy women do not have the pleasure of regularly seeing people like themselves being loved and wanted despite and perhaps because of their size, then it would come as no surprise that they would have trouble dreaming of experiencing that same pleasure for themselves as they are. So many of the television shows nowadays—*The Swan*, Khloe Kardashian's *Revenge Body*, episodes of *Maury*—focus on dramatic makeovers and weight loss in order to be attractive, acceptable, and, thus, loveable. Small wonder then why we have swaths of women who truly believe that no one will or can love them unless they look differently or that they will and can only be loved unless and until they lose weight. I know this to be true because for the longest time, I was one of those women.

For fat white actresses, white privilege seems to somewhat buffer them from the level of trolling Sidibe experiences. Melissa McCarthy is a plus-sized actress who has had her fair share of body shame heaped upon her (Busis), but there is rarely any mention of her race. Sonya Renee Taylor writes that the boldness that Amber Riley—a Black, plus-sized actress and former contestant on *Dancing with the Stars*—exhibits has not rewarded her as it has rewarded "Kirstie Alley, former Cheers star and [*Dancing With the Stars*] alum whose fatness was such a novelty in Hollywood that it garnered an entire HBO Series, *FatActress*."

Sidibe is not oblivious to the hate and the derision. She has said that people often ask her how and why she is so confident, as if amazed to see someone like her have such high self-esteem. She once said in reply:

> It's not easy. It's hard to get dressed up for award shows and red carpets when I know I will be made fun of because of my weight.[5] ... This is what I deal with every time I put on a dress. This is what I deal with every time someone takes a picture of me. Sometimes when I'm being interviewed by a fashion reporter, I can see it in her eyes, "How is she getting away with this? Why is she so confident? How does she deal with that body? Oh my God, I'm going to catch fat!" (qtd. in Vineyard)

In speaking about her confidence, she has also said the following: "[My confidence] came from me. One day I decided that I was beautiful, and so I carried out my life as if I was a beautiful girl. .... What matters is what you see. Your body is your temple, it's your home, and ... you must decorate it" (qtd. in Brown).

How then does one grate against arbitrary beauty standards? How does one deal with the unpopularity? Sidibe gives us a way forward in her Ms. Foundation gala speech: "I live my life, because I dare. I dare to show up when everyone else might hide their faces and hide their bodies in shame." (qtd. in Vineyard).

Being fat and Black may be persistently unpopular, but for Sidibe, I don't think it was ever about popularity. It was about being present. It's about being *seen*, despite not fitting the mould. It's about showing up, despite appearances. She dares to show up when people would rather she diet or die. I suppose that's all that life expects of us: show up, carve a path through the world's prejudices, and in the wake of your glory, leave everyone else alone to catch up and figure themselves out.

Endnotes

1. I use the word "fat" not in a pejorative sense but as merely a descriptor and the most neutral one that I can employ. Yes, it has its historical baggage, but it's better than saying "obese" (I discuss my discomfort with the word "obese" later) or using patronizing euphemisms, such as "curvy," "voluptuous," or "plus sized" (although I do use these latter terms interchangeable throughout the chapter).
2. While it is not the scope of this essay to discuss what it means to be obese, it should be noted that various communities and disciplines have their own definition of obesity. Gabourey Sidibe is arguably obese from a medical standpoint and from a Western hemisphere point of view, but the term obesity deserves to be problematized.
3. In his video response, Pastor Justin hinted at the same: "If I just saw her at face value, without knowing her, honestly I'd think this girl looks like she plays for the New York Giants.... Honestly, when I first saw her, it was like 'wow'" (Cox, "Would You Date").
4. The use of the word "bizarre" by Daniels alone demonstrates his own antifat beliefs. Even he is incredulous.
5. When she was vilified in the press for the white gown she wore to the Golden Globe awards in 2014, Sidibe took to Twitter and served her own dose of shade: "To people making mean comments about my GG pics, I most def cried about it on that private jet to my dream job last night. #jk" (qtd. in Uwumarogie).

Works Cited

Bossip Staff. "Gabby Sidibe Has a Man. Talk Amongst Yourselves." *Bossip*, 10 Jan. 2011, bossip.com/328973/gabby-sidibe-has-a-man-talk-amongst-yourselves12006. Accessed 5 Oct. 2020.

Brown, Laura. "Being Precious: Gabourey Sidibe." *Harpers Bazaar*, 7 Jan. 2010, www.harpersbazaar.com/celebrity/latest/news/a466/gabourey-sidibe-precious-interview-0210/. Accessed 5 Oct. 2020.

Busis, Hillary. "Melissa McCarthy Tackles Cruel Weight Comments." *CNN*, 14 June 2013, www.cnn.com/2013/06/13/showbiz/celebrity-news-gossip/melissa-mccarthy-weight-ew/index.html. Accessed 5 Oct. 2020.

Cox, Justin, "Pretty Women Are Overrated." *YouTube*, 8 Nov. 2009, www.youtube.com/watch?v=6ejPrae6P3M. Accessed 5 Oct. 2020.

Cox, Justin. "Would You Date the Girl from the Movie Precious." *YouTube*, 3 Apr. 2010, www.youtube.com/watch?v=hHhA_Kz9tS8. Accessed 5 Oct. 2020.

Hova, Trey. "Howard Stern Insults Gabourey Sidibe to the 10th Degree." *Vibe Magazine*, 10 Mar. 2010, www.vibe.com/2010/03/howard-stern-insults-gabourey-sidibe-10th-degree/. Accessed 5 Oct. 2020.

Jeffries, Stuart. "Meet Gabourey, the Star of Precious." *The Guardian*, 20 Jan. 2010, www.theguardian.com/film/2010/jan/20/gabby-sidibe-precious. Accessed 5 Oct. 2020.

Magowan, Margot. "Gabourey Sidibe Isn't Too Fat for Hollywood, She's Too Black." *San Francisco Gate Blog*, 14 Mar. 2010, blog.sfgate.com/mmagowan/2010/03/14/gabourey-sidibe-isnt-too-fat-for-hollywood-shes-too-black/. Accessed 5 Oct. 2020.

Mo'Nique. "Gabourey Sidibe." *Interview Magazine*, 17 Oct. 2009, www.interviewmagazine.com/film/gabourey-sidibe/#page2. Accessed 5 Oct. 2020.

Murphy, Tim. "Living the Life." *NewYorkMag*, 25 Sept. 2009, nymag.com/movies/profiles/59419/#ixzz0iGJDalya. Accessed 5 Oct. 2010.

Renee, Sonya. "Weight Stigma in Diverse Populations: Sonya Renee." *Binge Eating Disorders Association*, 23. Sept. 2013, bedaonline.com/wsaw2013/weight-stigma-diverse-populations-sonya-renee/#.UtT2E6E25KD. Accessed 5 Oct. 2020.

Stanley, Alessandra. "Wrought in Rhimes's Image: Viola Davis Plays Shonda Rhimes's Latest Tough Heroine." *New York Times*, 18. Sept. 2014, www.nytimes.com/2014/09/21/arts/television/viola-davis-plays-shonda-rhimess-latest-tough-heroine.htm. Accessed 5 Oct. 2020.

Taylor, Sonya Renee. "Weighting to Be Seen: Being Fat, Black and Invisible in Body Positivity." The Body is Not an Apology. 9 April 2017 https://thebodyisnotanapology.com/magazine/weighting-to-be-seen-being-fat-black-and-invisible-in-body-positivity/. Accessed 7 Nov. 2020.

Uwumarogie, Victoria. "Gabourey Sidibe Has Words for Those Who Slammed Her and Her Outfit at the Golden Globes." *Madame Noire*, 3 Jan. 2014, madamenoire.com/340226/gabourey-sidibe-golden-globes. Accessed 5 Oct. 2020.

Vineyard, Jennifer. "Read Gabourey Sidibe's Wonderful Speech from the Ms. Foundation Gala." *Vulture*, 2 May 2014, www.vulture.com/2014/05/read-gabourey-sidibes-ms-gala-speech.html?mid=twitter_vulturen. Accessed 5 Oct. 2020.

Wieselman, Jarett. "Gabourey Sidibe Refuses to Back Down." *Buzzfeed*, 11 Nov. 2015, www.buzzfeed.com/jarettwieselman/gabourey-sidibe-refuses-to-back-down#.fhV0ebjMlp. Accessed 5 Oct. 2020.

Williams, Mary Elizabeth. "Gabourey Sidibe Shuts Down the Trolls." *Salon*, 15 Jan. 2014, www.salon.com/2014/01/15/gabourey_sidibe_shuts_down_the_trolls/?upw. Accessed 5 Oct. 2020.

10.

She Says

Carrie Cox

Dedicated with love and thanksgiving for my miracle of a wee bee, Zoe Elyse, with whom I am honoured to dance, shimmy, and shake each and every day. She's my Gilmore Girl, through and through.

"Whenever we're hungry, we eat,"
Says She.
My Wee Bee.
I wonder...
Where did something
So fundamental
Seemingly so simple...
Where did it get lost?
(In the aisle next to the thigh masters and promises of thin?)
How can we even begin
To comprehend what our bodies truly need
If we can't just
Eat when we're hungry?
We talk calories
Weight
BMI
Piled high as the sky
Steeped in lies.
But why?
Why did food become the enemy?
Why do we wage a war against "obesity"

Instead of a war against hate?
When did "what I ate"
Become a reason for terrorizing
A body
Your body
Any body
All bodies
At the gym?
I don't even know where to begin
Except...

Friends, Romans, Countryfolk
Lend me your ears.
Listen and listen good
For just one moment
To Your Body.
It wants to:
Dance
Shimmy
Shake
Make the earth
Quake.
In celebration
In thanksgiving
In triumphant joy
For the miracle that
Your body knows
Deep in its bones
That it is.
(And Even if—
Especially if—
Voices both within
And without
Try to shout
that you are
Not A Miracle.
Listen to the miraculous beating
Of your heart.

Your body knows the truth.)
Your body
My body
Any body
All bodies
Are miracles.
Hungry for worship
From fingertip
To graceful hip.

And so...
Toss out the scales and measuring tapes.
They only inaccurately
Measure girth,
Not worth.
Instead...
Shatter the mirror
Watch it smash
Into a million tiny shards of glass.
False reflections no more
They rest,
Broken,
On the floor.
Waiting to be transformed into
Something New,
Something True.

And then...
And then
"Mama, let's dance,"
Says She,
My Wee Bee.

And then?
Even if—
Especially if—
You're not ready yet...
Pick up those tiny bits of broken glass.

Glue them, piece by piece
Bit by bit
Moment by moment
Day by Day
Into Something New,
Something True.
Make your own shining, sparkling
disco ball...
And dance the night away.

11.

The Elephant in the (Class)room

Christin L. Seher

My relationship with my body is complex, as it is for many. Growing up, I witnessed daily the hatred that my closest female friends and role models espoused for their bodies. I watched the people I cared most about lose parts of their identity, letting anorexia nervosa and obesity define them. However, as a youth, my own body was not a site of struggle; I was relatively thin and athletic; I rounded out in all the places society told me I should be.

Ironically, I became fat as I began to study nutrition as a graduate student. During my mid-twenties, never eating more healthfully or correctly, my body began to betray me. Using my newfound knowledge of nutrition and restrictive, controlled eating, I was able to contain (most of) the weight until I became pregnant with my son at the age of thirty, which also coincided with the beginning of my academic career teaching in a nutrition and dietetics program. Although my doctoral education prepared me extremely well for life as a faculty member, I was ill-prepared for how, through teaching, my body would be put on display daily, acting as proxy for my intellectual capabilities and professional competence.

I vividly remember the first day of the 2014-2015 academic year, getting dressed in the morning for my nutrition counselling and education skills course, and selecting a slightly form-fitting navy-blue dress from my closet to wear. Not one to usually dress up for class, I recall oscillating on the decision, thinking about the impression it would send to a new group of eager students. But it was going to be ninety degrees that August day, and I had recently bought, worn, and received several compliments on this particular dress at a conference presentation earlier in the month; still angry and embarrassed at how my midsection and breasts had changed shape so significantly since the birth of my son three and a half years before, I thought I had finally found a nice article of clothing I could wear with some level of confidence. As I walked into class—already self-conscious, but trying to project otherwise—I overheard one student comment to another, "Is that our professor?"

I wish I could say that it was my youthful appearance that prompted that comment, but I know better. At five foot six and two hundred pounds, my body was more reflective of one of the case study vignettes assigned to undergraduate dietetics students in their medical nutrition therapy courses than of the educators and preceptors who train future dietitians.

As I mature as a feminist scholar and teacher, I have come to realize the places where I diverge from the canon of my chosen profession form a chasm that, many times, seems impossible to bridge. For this reason, I often find myself reluctant to come out and disclose my credentials as a registered dietitian nutritionist to others. I do not want to hear about everything that particular person ate in the last week, the latest fad diet they are trying, their aunt with diabetes, or the rationale for their current food choices. I also do not want to explain why I chose this profession, when, on the surface, my philosophy is so divergent from mainstream dietetics. At least, that is what I tell myself. Deep down, I also know a large part of why I do not outwardly identify to others as a dietitian is because I want to avoid the dissonance produced, which visibly registers in others, upon hearing my disciplinary expertise and comparing the body that contains it.

In the classroom, I do not have that luxury. My body betrays me each and every time I stand in front of an audience. Similar to how Judith Butler describes gender, teaching is "a performance, *a stylized repetition of acts*" (519). And it is clear that my body does not fit the role. As such, upon meeting each new group of students, I grow more and more cognizant of the ways in which I must prove myself a worthy professor—ways in which my thin female colleagues do not. This critical gaze comes from more than my students; it is felt from colleagues in other disciplines, from community collaborators, other health professionals, and from parents I meet as well. It also comes from within. Through my professional socialization into dietetics, I have internalized the fatphobia and body hatred that fuels a large part of the work that dietitians do (but that is a paper for another time). Working towards body acceptance is difficult, however much desired, while encumbered in a discipline that reifies in true Foucauldian fashion discourses of discipline, surveillance, and regulation surrounding food and the body in Western culture.

The topic of fat bodies in the classroom has received relatively little exploration in the scholarly literature, despite both the increasing field of fat studies and the wide acknowledgment by critical pedagogues, such as bell hooks, that bodies do matter to the teaching environment. Christina Fisanick, writing about her own experience as a fat professor, notes how fat instructors stand in opposition to the normative "professor body"—that of a white, middle-class, able-bodied, heterosexual, thin male (239)—and that image forms the ideal against which they are judged by students and colleagues. Those who do not fit this archetype, therefore, must combat both the "neoliberal biopolitics that couples control and deservingness and deems the improperly embodied subject as a problem for the broader social body" (Guthman 1126) and the stereotype that they are lazy, gluttonous, weak-willed, uneducated, and morally lacking—hardly the image of a university professor. As a dietetics educator, this normative professor ideal is further bound by cultural and disciplinary notions of what a dietitian is and what she should look like, as body size and shape are not only tied to judgments of personal morality and character but to professional competence as well.

Therefore, those who argue that bodies don't matter—that a Cartesian split between the mind and body is a natural binary for a university classroom seeking enlightenment—are ignoring the reality that the body has, as Fisanick writes, "powerful effects and possibilities in the classroom" (246). Yofi Tirosh, similarly, likens her body size as an instructor to "an expressive force" (268), one that is shielded in discourse yet open to interrogation. This examination, Tirosh explains, involves coming out of the "fat closet" (as first described by Sedgwick 72), acknowledging the negative cultural values assigned to oneself, based upon body size, and, thus, opening the body as well as the discourses surrounding it up to interrogation.

Like the women above, one way I have come to deal with the uncomfortable discrepancy between my mind and body is by learning to intentionally use my body in the classroom as a pedagogical tool, placing it in a precarious, vulnerable, and often demoralizing position. Through the incorporation of feminist pedagogy, my dietetics classroom becomes a place to name, contest, and "talk back"—however briefly—to a profession and broader society that constructs and perpetuates neoliberal discourse linking morality and worth to manifestations of the body (Hoverd; Guthman). I do this by introducing future nutrition professionals to such topics as thin privilege, body acceptance movements, and the health at every size counselling approach (Aphramor and Bacon; Bacon) by asking them to consider obesity discourse and how health professionals speak of fatness and its etiology and by requiring them to critically examine their relationship with food and their own bodies through reflective writing exercises. All the while, I embody the fatness that dietetics as a profession is so focused upon combatting.

In essence, through course discussion, I intentionally and repeatedly come out to my students as a fat dietitian. I address head on the elephant in the room that is present whether I want it to be or not and ask my students to consider what assumptions could be made about me, as a person of size, by a healthcare practitioner. After the initial uncomfortableness, a rich discussion is typically had about the assumptions we as dietitians project on our patients—often labelling them as lazy, noncompliant, and uneducated—and the potential problems with a patient-counsellor relationship built upon that kind of foundation. I also ask them to consider how patients might be reading their bodies as well and ask them to think about how their identities—as predominantly thin, white, able-bodied, heterosexual, and middle-class women—matter in the work they want to do. I ask students to examine, via autobiographical writing, how their health status and body size/shape intersects with their lived experiences to contribute to their desire to study dietetics and to help others with their own nutrition. I also introduce them to the idea of healthism[1] (Greenhalgh and Wessely 200; Tirhas 56) as a moral and political ideology that shapes the aims of our profession and, more acutely, the motivations of the food, diet, and weight-loss industries.

Of course, these kinds of pedagogical exercises must be approached with caution and come only after substantial reflection on the part of an instructor to fully articulate their pedagogical purpose. More than once, I have found myself contemplating if the reason I include these topics into the courses I teach is personal—as Tirosh also questions—as a "means for 'justifying' my deviance" from normative body ideals (276). I also have questioned (more than once) if my pedagogical aims are worth the risk as a professor not protected by tenure. Part of the reason I include these topics, certainly, stems from my subjectivities, having experienced the same kind of disenfranchisement that many fat individuals do. More importantly, however, I am a feminist teacher. I want my students to begin to question the social construction of fatness, how the profession of dietetics contributes to this construction, and how their assumptions as practitioners about the patients they work with may affect the healthcare they deliver. I want students to hear the voices of fat individuals in society and consider how those realities may play a role in their weight loss attempts, successes and barriers, or motivate a patient's journey towards body acceptance. I want dietetics students, such as those in other disciplines, to train their inner critic and cultivate the kind of critical thinking skills they need to evaluate, critique, and challenge the assumptions of contemporary dietetics practice. As a profession striving towards cultural humility, I believe this is a crucial skill to foster in novice dietitians—the desire to be a reflexive practitioner, able to authentically relate to diverse individuals and be cognizant of how one's own belief structure affects the way that they work.

So where do I go next?

The literature calls for further scrutiny into the ways in which professors' bodies shape their design and delivery of class content and the way in which such content is received by students (Watkins, Farrell, and Hugmeyer 11). By some accounts (Fisanick 248), it seems as though being fat, while teaching about perspectives on fatness, lends credibility and goes further in being able to create a safe space for students to examine fat discrimination. I cannot know for certain whether or not I would have arrived at the desire to push my students' thinking on this topic had I not gained weight myself; what I do know for certain is that body size is only one aspect of identity with which I ask my students to engage. Long before I considered incorporating discussions on body size, I framed my classroom as a liberatory space, including pedagogical exercises (e.g., poverty simulations, ally training, and reflexive writing assignments) in the curriculum to expand critical consciousness and build reflexive practice. In my opinion, it was only a matter of time, thin or fat, before I arrived in this space.

Another topic lending itself to further examination is the role of pedagogy in pushing students to examine their own relationship with their bodies (Wakins, Farrell, and Hugmeyer 12). Since the introduction of these topics in my courses, I have seen safe spaces created for students to disclose their personal struggles with weight and nutrition, which is important for dietitians, in particular, who overwhelmingly report a history of eating disorders, weight struggles, and disordered eating patterns (Arroyo et. al 126; Drummond and Hare 86; Houston, Bassler and Anderson 724). In a way, as Bacon (1) suggests, as a successful, highly-educated dietetics professor, I have the potential to be a powerful role model for my students as they work through the complicated dynamics that brought them to study dietetics. In order to do that, there is a lot of work I still need to do first. In addition, I wrestle with the notion that despite having a background in food and nutrition, I am not trained as a psychotherapist and, thus, cannot provide the kind of support students may need in navigating their body acceptance journey.

The best I can do at this point is keep pushing in hopes of furthering this important conversation. I made the decision to author this chapter publicly, despite risk and vulnerability, in the hopes that it sparks a much-needed conversation among those of us educating future health professionals. As I negotiate this uncomfortable terrain, I am grateful for my feminist epistemology, as it provides the language and framework from which to draw upon in navigating an emotionally draining and, at times, openly hostile climate where I am subject to microaggressions daily based upon my body size. Bodies can and do matter both in the delivery and receptivity of course material, and not addressing the elephant in the (class)room can, at times, derail the powerful possibilities bodies hold for the pedagogical aims of the classroom.

Endnotes

1. "Healthism" as defined by Trisha Greenhalgh and Simon Wessely reflects how "the beliefs, behaviour, and expectations of the articulate, health-aware, and information-rich middle classes" (197) frame health as a moral imperative and the result of a collective of individual decisions.

Works Cited

Arroyo, Marta, et al. "Prevalence and Magnitude of Body Weight and Image Dissatisfaction among Women in Dietetics Majors." *Archivos LatinoAmericanos De Nutrición*, vol. 60, no. 2, 2010, pp. 126-32.

Aphramor, Lucy, and Linda Bacon. *Body Respect: What Conventional Health Books Get Wrong, Leave Out, and Just Plain Fail to Understand about Weight*. BenBella Books, 2014.

Bacon, Linda. *Health at Every Size: The Surprising Truth about Your Weight*. BenBella Books, 2008.

Butler, Judith. "Performative Acts and Gender Constitution: An Essay in Phenomenology and Feminist Theory." *Theatre Journal*, vol. 40, no. 4, 1988, pp. 519-31.

Drummond, Dianne, and M. Suzanne Hare. "Dietitians and Eating Disorders: An International Issue." *Perspectives in Practice*, vol. 73, no. 2, 2012, pp. 86-90.

Fisanick, Christina. "'They Are Weighted with Authority': Fat Female Professors in Academic and Popular Cultures." *Feminist Teacher*, vol. 17, no. 3, 2007, pp. 237-55.

Greenhalgh, Trisha and Simon Wessely. "'Health for Me': A Sociocultural Analysis of Healthism in the Middle Classes." *British Medical Bulletin*, vol. 69, 2004, pp. 197-213.

Guthman, Julie. "Teaching the Politics of Obesity: Insights into Neoliberal Embodiment and Contemporary Biopolitics." *Antipode*, vol. 41, no. 5, 2009, pp. 1110-33.

hooks, bell. *Teaching to Transgress: Education as the Practice of Freedom*. Routledge, 1994.

Houston, Cheryl, Eunice Bassler, and Jean Anderson. "Eating Disorders among Dietetics Students: An Educator's Dilemma." *Journal of the American Dietetic Association*, vol. 108, no. 4, 2008, pp. 722-24.

Sedgwick, Eve Kosofsky. *Epistemology of the Closet*. University of California Press, 1990.

Tirhas, Cristina. "The Healthist Ideology: Towards a New Form of Health Awareness in the Contemporary Lifestyle?" *Studia Ubb. Philosophia*, vol. 57, no. 3, 2012, pp. 55-70.

Tirosh, Yofi. "Weighty Speech: Addressing Body Size in the Classroom." *The Review of Education, Pedagogy, and Cultural Studies*, vol. 28, 2006, pp. 267-79.

Watkins, Patti, Amy Farrelland, and Andrea Doyle Hugmeyer. "Teaching Fat Studies: From Conception to Reception." *Fat Studies*, vol. 1, no. 2, pp. 180-94.

12.

"Your Wheelchair Is So Slim": A Meditation on the Social Enactment of Beauty and Disability

Samantha Walsh

The Desire to Be Beautiful

"Your wheelchair is so thin." These were the off-handed remarks of a beautician. However, these words and the phrases that followed gave me pause both personally and academically. This comment was the impetus for the following chapter.

The desire to be understood as beautiful is a desire that I cannot remember being without. I remember wanting to be understood as beautiful as a young girl; now as a full-fledged adult, the desire has not left me. However, my definition of beauty has shifted as I have grown. My current identity is that of a scholar, disability rights activist, woman, and wheelchair user. My disability has often been treated as something that mars or disrupts my beauty. I have had individuals abruptly tell me that I am too pretty to use a wheelchair or that my beauty was a waste, since I am disabled. Additionally, and perhaps most relevant to the topic of this anthology, although I cannot place the origin of this idea, I have often felt that it was compulsory that if my beauty was confounded by my disability, the least I could do to comply with normative body expectations was to try and be as thin as possible. While as a child this notion was quite disturbing, as a sociologist, this tension between beauty, disability, and body size has become an opportunity for curiosity. From an academic perspective, I have become interested in the taken for granted social position of beauty (specifically in Western society) and how it interacts with disability and gender.

Beauty as a Cultural Construct

This chapter will focus on the placement of beauty and disability within society through an analysis of a conversation I had with a beauty service provider in her salon. This conversation provided an opportunity to interrogate this social dyad of beauty and disability through three distinct themes. First, the beautician suggested that there is never a reason "not to be feminine"; the beautician understood feminine as being synonymous with being thin. Second, she endorsed a sense of compulsory normative behaviour to fit in, and in doing this, from her words, an understanding of those who do not fit in emerged as tragic or deviant. Third, her narrative told me a day spa or beauty salon is an unlikely place for disability to be seen.

To begin, the role of beauty within contemporary society must first be contextualized. For the purposes of this chapter and the analysis of my conversation with the beautician, I will be discussing beauty as it relates to those understood as women. The voice of culture is written on our bodies. To that end, the voice of dominant Western society writes on the bodies of women that hierarchy and male dominance must be maintained. The voice of our culture privileges the normative white male heterosexual body. It privileges the performance that is male heteronormative enactment. Debra Gimlin explicates the concept of the body as a medium of culture: "It is the surface on which prevailing rules of a culture are written. The shared attitudes and practices of social groups are played out at the level of the body, revealing cultural notions of distinctions ... cultural rules are not only revealed through the body; they also shape the way the body performs and appears (3).

Gimlin's notion is useful in identifying the social production that beauty creates. To that end, the work of Judith Butler further confirms not only that the beautification of the body is a function of social control but also that gender is an enactment through which social status is allocated. Butler's work in unpacking the social performance of gender unsettles the notion that the hallmarks of the body are innate. Her work allows for the discussion of gender performance as an expression rather than a preexisting identity. Butler's work unsettles in-born notions of the body and creates space for the discussion of social performance. She reminds us that "There is no gender identity behind the expressions of gender ... identity is performatively constituted by the very 'expressions' that are said to be its results" (25). Butler unpacks the notions that gender and embodiment are innate. She contends that the enactment of gender is reinforced by the acceptance and access people gain into society.

Making Beauty

Both the notion of the body as a cultural medium, the concept of performativity, and the role beauty plays in women's access to resources become useful in theorizing the conversation between me and the beautician. The conversation arose out of the beautician telling me about another client who also uses a wheelchair. She contrasted my embodiment with the other woman by saying, "Your wheelchair is so slim. My other client has a big bulky wheelchair." Unsure of how to answer, I said "Umm thank you?" She went on to explain that she did not understand why one would use such a "big heavy" wheelchair when, in contrast, mine was so "slim and feminine." In this conversation, the voice of the beautician became the dominant voice of our shared culture. She ascribed that much like a woman is expected to be slim and feminine, so too should that woman's wheelchair. She praised me for having a wheelchair she could barely see, one that made few marks on the doors or noise in a room. She understood my wheelchair as blending in, ascribing it a subordinate character. She was commending me for selecting a wheelchair that ironically embodied the same sort of characteristics women are praised for having within the dominant culture. The voice of our culture was so powerful that it was writing on me and also my wheelchair. Interestingly, in contrast, I am not often understood as a thin woman. In my personal and professional life, I am often criticized for being too loud or in the way. The explicit and implicit message is often that I should do more to curb my verbose presence. The beautician's compliment was one that brought up interesting tensions between disability and beauty but also reaffirmed Western cultural ideas that women like me should make themselves small.

Her comment of praise for my having a wheelchair that she understood as not being that noticeable also speaks to the way disability is understood through the dominant cultural lens. She found my wheelchair to be pleasing, as she could not see it; therefore, it did not remind her of disability.

I interjected that a wheelchair is a very personal selection and that aesthetics are often sacrificed for functionality or are understood as superfluous and dismissed by the service provider or vender. In my case, my wheelchair was the sum of many other social intersectionalities and was likely the product of existing in an environment where everyone involved understood disability as a valid embodiment.

The beautician responded with "But even your body looks normal. I think this woman could do more to look better."

Women's Bodies and the Compulsory Expectation of Beauty

The cultural voice demands the woman's body be improved. Sandra Bartky further explains this cultural paradigm:

> A woman's face must be made up, that is to say, made over, and so must her body: she is ten pounds overweight; her lips must be made more kissable; her complexion dewier; her eyes more mysterious. The "art" of make-up is the art of disguise, but this presupposes that a woman's face, unpainted, is defective. Soap and water, a shave, and routine attention to hygiene may be enough for *him*; for *her* they are not. (71)

Bartky's analysis of the cultural paradigm of women's bodies as being defective denotes why it was plausible for the beautician to feel the other woman should be doing more to be beautiful. It was treated as self-evident that this woman should be doing more to enact the embodiment our culture favours. Furthermore, the beautician associated beauty with the normalcy of my body; I was being praised for my act of erasing difference. Neither my body nor my wheelchair reminded her of disability. Disability is a concept that the mainstream culture finds troubling; just as there is a compulsion to improve or beautify the woman's body, there is a compulsion to normalize the disabled body. Rosemarie Garland-Thomson explicates this concept:

> Many parallels exist between the social meanings attributed to female bodies and those assigned to disabled bodies. Both the female and the disabled body are cast as deviant and inferior; both are excluded from full participation in public as well as economic life; both are defined in opposition to a norm that is assumed to possess natural physical superiority. (19)

In the salon, captured within the interactions between me and this beautician, the writings of Garland-Thomson came to life. The (other) woman in question was understood as deviant for not correctly enacting beauty and also for being unable and/or unwilling to hide the visual hallmarks of a disability she wore.

The beautician continued to question and scrutinize why this woman would not make herself more beautiful. Thinking out loud, she said "Maybe she can't get a smaller wheelchair? Maybe she's severely disabled? Do you think that's the issue?" The inference of needing a smaller wheelchair to be beautiful is again a notion that disability must be minimized to be beautiful. The attempt to quantify this woman's disability as being severe as a justification for not being beautiful socially produces the notion that for beauty and disability to exist, the disability must be minimal, and the beauty must be exceptional. Furthermore, it is treated as self-evident that it is not a choice or a purposeful act for the individual to construct herself visually as she does. The woman wearing a wheelchair is understood through the dominant voice as being subjugated by the intersection of disabled within her identity. Her disability is understood by the voice of our culture (and literally the voice of the beautician) as detracting from her ability to perform beauty. At no point is the disabled woman understood as purposely manifesting her look or having some sort of agency in her performance. She is understood as a pliable entity who bends under the weight of the disability. Moreover, disability is not entertained as something that may enhance or be a positive asset to her character. It is always understood as a hindrance to her beauty. Her disability becomes something that must be overcome in order to be beautiful.

The discussion between me and the beautician suggests to me that the beautician understands me as someone who has minimized their disability and can, therefore, be understood as beautiful. This sentiment is fraught with the tension of my own lived narrative in juxtaposition to the dominant understanding of disability. Although I am pleased to be understood as a social commodity that can both be desirable and of value, I am disheartened by the statement that my disability must be minimized to be understood as desirable and valuable. I understand the social position of women being social commodities to be problematic but struggle to find recourse. The tension mounts as I am presented with the location that I am a social product and am expected to do something with my body both to minimize my disability and to perform my gender. The beautician has explained that beauty is to be understood in the minimization or erasure of disability. That a failure to enact this is only understood as a manifestation of deviance or personal tragedy. The mainstream cannot fathom that there is any sort of alternative to enacting beauty. Beauty is understood in the context of the mainstream and enacted within the microcosm of my interaction with the beautician as being the absence of disability and the hyperperformance of mainstream hallmarks of femininity. To be beautiful is to be understood as normal. Garland-Thomson takes up this interaction of normal being understood as beautiful in her theorizing of the concept of the term "normate":

> The term normate usefully designates the social figure through which people can represent themselves as definitive human beings. Normate, then, is the constructed identity of those who, by way of the bodily configurations and cultural capital they assume, can step into a position of authority and wield the power it grants them. If one attempts to define the normate position by peeling away all the marked traits within the social order at this historical moment, what emerges is a very narrowly defined profile that describes only a minority of actual people. (8)

Garland-Thomson's concept of "normate," thus, exposes the falseness of beauty. She illustrates that only a small portion of people can be understood as existing within normate culture. Everyone who does not must then socially produce a sense of being normal. The conversation between me and the beautician is a manifestation of this cultural need to socially produce normalcy, as the beautician understands the normal body to represent the existence of beauty while disability represents a disruption of the normal body. The disabled body exists on the margins of beauty. The beautician's construction of beauty as a microcosm of the mainstream understanding of beauty infers that disability does not exist with beauty. The two cannot exist in the same space, the same body, the same perception. This relationship between disability and beauty is socially produced within not only our words and interactions but also the physical space we inhabit.

The room we (the beautician and I) are in is accessible-ish. My wheelchair fits through the door with no scuffs and no scratches, but this other wheeled woman's wheelchair and conversely her body do not fit in the space, and she is not welcome. She is understood as being outside the realm of what can be made beautiful. Although the beautician must serve her, it is done so with a sense of pity and tragedy that her body exists in a state that is beyond repair. She may receive beauty services and subscribe to the same sort of beautification work as women who are understood as able-bodied, but she cannot achieve beauty, as beauty is produced in the absence of disability. This construction of beauty as being the absence of disability is prevalent in the physical space of the salon and other places of beauty ritual. It exists within our interactions and permeates our individual understandings of beauty. The culture of beauty is a heavy and suffocating one.

The words of the beautician are the vocal manifestations of a culture that maintains and reenforces gender norms, compulsory heterosexuality, and a compulsory embodiment. I am there because it is my understanding that I must look a certain way to be understood as a social commodity and to be understood as valid within my society. I disagree with the structure and its organization, but I am unable to escape the heavy beauty culture. The understanding that disability does not exist within beauty is reproduced inside the salon but also outside of it. I, apparently a learned academic, still continue to interact with rituals of beauty and purchase services from someone who essentially verbally violates the validity of my embodiment, all in the name of achieving beauty.

In the context of contemporary society, beauty is understood as a tool for women to gain access to power structures and resources, as Naomi Wolf reminds us:

> Women learned to crave "beauty" in its contemporary form because we were learning at the same time that the feminist struggle was going to be much harder than we had realized. The ideology of "beauty" was a shortcut promise to agitating women, a historical placebo—that we could be confident, valued, heard out, respected, and make demands without fear. (In fact, it is doubtful whether "beauty" is the real desire at all; women may

> want "beauty" that we can forget about the whole damn thing. Most women, in their guts, would probably rather be, given the choice, a sexual, courageous self, than a beautiful generic other. (282)

Although the commodification of women through beauty is problematic in general, the notion that beauty exists in the absence of disability is fraught with social repercussions. If beauty is the tool that women can use to gain access into society and disability negates this, disability then becomes something to be avoided, minimized, and erased at all costs. Disability then becomes something that is not welcome in our society. If disability must be minimized or erased for things to be beautiful, then there becomes no space to celebrate, theorize, or live disability. Disability becomes something that must be rehabilitated, cured, erased, trivialized, and removed. In rethinking beauty and why "your wheelchair is so slim" is a compliment, we must also rethink the place of disability in our greater contemporary society. By rethinking disability, we make space both literally and figuratively for the woman riding the bulky wheelchair, an alternative to mainstream beauty construction, a reappropriation of gender norms, and a more inclusive notion of beauty.

Conclusion

In this recreation of beauty, we can make space and question the role of beauty in general and the common sense understanding of disability. In this space, we can expose the look we are obsessed with as a contemporary culture and understand it as far more than a look. We can begin to see it as the manifestation of a production of gender performance, the visual hallmarks of social capital written on our bodies, and representative of how and where we place disability as a contemporary society. The look is the metaphorical map of our culture composed on our bodies. It is my hope this map will not be simply consumed but rather taken up as an opportunity to question and reflect on the spaces in which we exist.

Works Cited

Bartky, S. L. *Femininity and Domination: Studies in the Phenomenology of Domination*. Routledge, 1990.

Butler, Judith. *Gender Trouble: Feminism and the Subversion of Identity*. Routledge, 2011.

Garland-Thomson, Rosemarie. *Extraordinary Bodies: Figuring Physical Disability in American Culture and Literature*. Columbia University Press, 1997.

Gimlin, Debra. *Body Work: Beauty and Self-Image in American Culture*. University of California Press, 2002.

Wolf, Naomi. *The Beauty Myth: How images of Beauty Are Used against Women*. Random House, 2013.

13.

My Body Is My Business

Liis Windischmann

He told me to stand on the giant scale in the middle of the modelling agency reception area. My head was screaming no. My heart was screaming no. But I found my seventeen-year-old self getting up on that scale. "What did you eat today?" the agent asked in an accusatory tone. I remember mumbling something about my healthy breakfast and my snack... a cranberry muffin. It's interesting the facts we remember decades later.

"No more cranberry muffins for you!" he bellowed as he wagged his finger in my face. I felt every set of eyes in the small room staring at me getting scolded. "And start dieting and come back weekly for weigh-ins." I don't recall saying a word. I may have grunted. I shuffled out feeling stung. I was too mad at myself for not having walked right out of that agency. Too mad for getting on that scale. Too mad for letting someone tell me there was something wrong with my healthy body. Too mad I didn't say something. Anything. I never went back.

After visiting another agency and having all my so-called flaws pointed out, along with being told to yet again lose weight, I gave up my pipe dream of becoming a model. At about 130 pounds and almost six feet tall, I was a healthy and active teenager. I was the kid on every school sports team who loved to work out for the sheer thrill of doing so. My mom made us eat our veggies and have salad every night. I craved fruits and vegetables and regularly requested Brussel sprouts. I knew I was more than just okay. I knew my body was capable, healthy, athletic, and strong.

I went off to university and got my degree and some hips, too. By then I was a size fourteen. Soon after graduating, I was walking through a mall in Toronto and was stopped by a model scout. I can still remember her startled face as I rebuffed her in a one-way conversation after asking me if I wanted to become a model.

"I know you want me to lose weight." (Insert slight roll of my eyes here.)

"No thank you. "(I am not going there with you lady.)

"I am not interested." (I have so heard this before.)

Eventually, after I let her get a word in edgewise, she replied, "I don't want you to lose a pound." I stared at her waiting for the sales pitch punchline—the offer of expensive modelling classes. There had to be a catch. "Have you ever heard of plus-size modelling?" I had not.

This was the early 1990s, and the industry was in its infancy. The internet hadn't taken off yet, and there was no social media, websites, or bloggers. I rarely looked at newspaper flyers. I thought all models were skinny because every woman in every magazine I ever opened was the same small size and the agencies I had visited years before had confirmed this.

"So, you mean I can model exactly the way I am? I don't have to lose a pound?"

"Yes."

"Well, now you have my interest. Please tell me more."

And that is how my twenty-three-year career started in plus-size fashion.

When you start your career with a solid foundation—one in which you feel true to the core of your being, and your mind, body, and soul scream YES!—life really is delicious. I don't know many who can say that when they show up for work, they and their bodies feel honoured. Every time I was on set, in a fashion show, on television, or in a campaign, I felt honoured to represent many girls and women who never saw themselves in fashion.

As a model, there is an intimacy and a sense of comfort that develops when you, whether regularly appearing on television or in a print ad, are in essence invited into someone's home on their television screen or in photos placed on the family's kitchen table. "You're the _______ girl!" women would often exclaim when we met in person after having seen me regularly on Cityline's Fashion Friday segments or as the face of a popular brand. The comments were often the same: "Thank you. You look like me. When I see you, I feel included in fashion. I have a better idea of what an outfit may actually look like on my body. You looked so confident in that outfit I feel like I can wear it too!"

Whenever I walked in a fashion show, I was often the only model over a size two, sometimes walking the runway with a couple other plus-size models. The crowd would react loudly. I knew they were seeing themselves up there. I knew they felt included. Being a plus-size model wasn't just a job. My curvy body was a statement of inclusiveness.

My body in all its curviness allowed me a career travelling the world exploring countries and cultures I never would have seen otherwise. It took me to the Sahara Desert of Africa, the pink-sand beaches of the Caribbean, the vineyards, marinas, and mountains of Europe, and the markets across North America. My curves allowed me to wander the cobblestone streets of European cities, attempting conversations with amused locals in broken German and French. I have lived in Toronto, New York, Chicago, and Miami. And my body—the body the model scout told me was just perfect without losing a pound—made me money to make all these adventures possible; it kept a roof over my head and provided a happy life.

Whereas many in society would deem extra curves a curse, I saw my voluptuous frame as a means of travelling the world with a beautiful message of body love that opened up positivity and conversations. I refused to attend any weight-loss castings or be submitted for any diet-related job, and trust me, they paid well. I made a point of having this noted on every chart for every agency I worked for. A new booker not familiar with my chart once excitedly called to tell me I had a strong chance of securing a booking for a weight-loss company—a thirty thousand dollar job. I told her to remove me from the running. She was stunned and kept trying to get me to change my mind. Could I have used the money? Absolutely! But the price I would have had to pay would have been too high. And my body had been too good to me to turn on it, to diminish its value, and to cash it in for a campaign that did not resonate with my soul's purpose on this planet.

Although I didn't realize it at the time, in 2011, I was commencing the ultimate body-love journey. I had discovered the joy of jogging and was getting ready for my first five kilometre race. After months of gasping, I was finally finding my groove and discovering that elusive runners' high I had always heard about. It was quite magical and exciting until one day, a few minutes into my run, I ran out of energy and literally flew off the end of the treadmill into the wall. I did not know it at the time, but that would be my very last workout, my very last run. My health began plummeting rapidly. Several months later, I was diagnosed with Hashimoto's, an autoimmune thyroid dis-ease[1] in which the autoimmune system mistakenly attacks the thyroid. It zapped me of all energy, caused my hair to fall out in chunks, and turned my world upside down.

I kept pushing on and worked through increasing pain, growing health problems, and mind fog. My size-sixteen, plus-sized body allowed me to model and do television appearances as an on-air spokesperson talking about plus-size fashion. All my years of improv training mixed with modelling were coming into play as I did live television. It was my sweet spot, and I loved it. But I was working so hard to look normal all the time in public while a multitude of health problems kept developing. My body was talking to me, pleading with me. I just wasn't processing the information.

In September of 2013, I had the honour of receiving a body image award from the Body Confidence Canada Awards. On a night in which I should have been celebrating all my body had allowed me to do over a long career, while the speeches took place, I felt both my body and mind imploding. The room started to spin. I got extremely clammy and felt like I was going to pass out. Everything felt off in a way my body had never experienced before. I started to sigh really loudly; it sounded exasperated, rude, and loud. I remember getting a few quizzical looks as I quickly tried to leave at the end of the night. After only consuming water, I found myself stumbling to my car. I removed my high heels and walked barefoot on the concrete. As I sat in my car blasting the air conditioning, I knew something was very wrong with my body and my brain.

Within two weeks, I was having severe trouble walking, talking, and using my hands. I could not get a fork to my mouth without stabbing myself in the face. I stopped eating anything with a spoon because I would drop the food on me or burn myself with hot soup. Soon I couldn't open cans or jars anymore. I could not do up a button, my shoelaces, or a necklace. My mind felt like it was disintegrating. The way my body and brain were rapidly declining, I thought I was developing dementia and would be in a nursing home. I was in a complete panic. It wasn't just my body that was crumbling; my entire world was as well.

I was very fortunate to get a diagnosis within months of gluten ataxia, a rare dis-ease in which gluten causes an autoimmune reaction against cells in the cerebellum, the section of the brain in charge of motor skills. Much of the time I looked and sounded like I was drunk. Like a mother protecting her child, all I wanted to do was shower my body with love. Send it all the energy it needed in any form it needed it. Hold it and say, "I've got you. Everything is going to be okay. I love you no matter what." And one day I did just that. Racked in pain and sobbing, I cradled my body and said out loud, "Be whatever size you need to be. Be a four. Be a fourteen. Be a twenty-four. Pick a size that lets you run around and be pain free. It doesn't matter to me."

It was in that moment I realized how deep my body love ran. How deep the level of appreciation was for my body that had carried me around countries, had put food on my table, paid my mortgage, and was literally woven into the fabric of my life. It had treated me so well, and I just wanted to take care of it, fix it, make it better.

When you have been in daily pain for years, you will do whatever it takes to feel well. I sent my incredible body—my body that had made my career, my world, and my life so beautiful—all the love in the world. I nourished it every way I knew how, through self-love, meditation, holistic healing, low-stress living, Qigong, supplements—you name it. And most importantly, I ate the healthiest way I could according to the research I did and with my health team's advice, which involved adopting a gluten-free and Paleo way of eating. I didn't eat less, and I didn't go on a diet. I just ate differently, cutting out processed and inflammatory foods; I cooked and baked more, feeding my body different fuel. My motto became "Every meal is a gift to heal." Within two weeks of adopting the Paleo lifestyle, the severe pain I had felt daily for years vanished. I wept on my knees in gratitude.

My celebrations became about regaining my dexterity and mobility and being able to have the strength to hug people and shake their hands, being able to type, think and create again. I rejoiced in being able to stave off buying a mobility scooter. When years of daily nausea vanished, I wept again. Those tears of gratitude were the sweetest tears I had ever cried.

When almost all the comments I received about my physical changes simply revolved around the fact that I had lost weight and my shape had dramatically changed and, thus, I looked amazing, it stunned me to the core of my being. I became highly protective of my body. I loved my body whether it was a plus-size sixteen or a straight-size twelve, the two ends of my size spectrum or any size in between or above for that matter. My curvy body at any size had provided a wonderful career and a beautiful life; it had now done everything in its power to protect me on a long health journey. It was too important and precious to be cast aside with casual comments.

My body has been intertwined with my career for twenty-three years. No matter what it looks like or what size my dress label reads, or where my future levels of ability rest, or what the scale at the doctor's office says I weigh, I am grateful, and I am proud. The gifts I have received through my body will fuel my career of body love for the rest of my life.

After several years of dis-ease, it feels as though I am coming out of a long slumber and trying to catch up with the rest of the world. As I try to redefine myself in the newness, I know my body and its story will always be a part of my career. Its experiences hold valuable information for others and lessons worth sharing—love worth sharing.

And if I could go back to speak with my seventeen-year-old self, I would tell her not to be angry. I would tell her that stepping off that scale and walking away was bravery in motion. It was an experience and decision that would become one of her life's greatest gifts and would shape her future through draping it in confidence and happiness. I would tell her that her beautiful body, at any size, thanks her through all time and space.

Endnotes

1. Like many who practice holistic health, I use the term "dis-ease" versus disease. The hyphenation is used with the intention of not empowering a particular health issue but rather placing the emphasis on the ability to get back from a state of imbalance to a state of ease.

14.

On Learning Self-Love: How One Curvy, Disabled Brown Femme Navigates the Body as a Site of Daily Struggle of Living with/in Pain

Anoop Kaur

When I remember to breathe, my body tells me where I need to start. But how does my breath know my body? And my body, my breath? It seems like knowing one's body, along with each exhale, is a self-explanatory act. But, for me, it's quite the opposite. Most days, I feel like both my breath and my body are unknown to me in the most silent and secret of ways. So how do I start back at the beginning; to unlearn the shame and hatred that surrounds my body, my femmeness,[1] and my disability? Although I remember and sometimes forget, I always start back at the same place: I lace up my shoes and I start running.

2017 and 27. I've often been told that my baby face does not match my age. But a quiet truth is that my body and heart feel so very old. Since I can remember, my body has been a site of daily struggle—of race, of blood, of belonging, and never belonging. And, as such, I cannot remember a time when I haven't been weighed down by body labour that is gendered, raced, classed, and disabled. Existing in a body that betrays me regularly has been ever constant, along with a nagging hunger I can never satisfy. So, throughout the years, I have been struggling to remind myself that my body is mine. But in this slow process of reminders, I have continued to fail in grasping the magic that is my body in the palms of my hands. I have been unable to swallow this magic whole to sustain me. But this is the way that shame shapes my Brown disabled femme body. This is the way that shame has morphed my body into something that is completely unrecognizable to the self, until the peeking of bones surface like dents in white hospital sheets.

To be clear, the rejection of my Brown blossoming body when I was nine was not the rejection of my femme(inity) but of growth and change. As a child I hated change, as it was symbolic of my obvious difference. How could I fit in with skin that was not porcelain white, with D cup adolescent breasts, thick thighs, and an Arabic name that never translates to white tongues? These aspects of myself were signifiers of my difference, of my unbelonging, and of my otherness. And so, growing up racialized, I always longed to reinvent myself anew, and through my eating disorder, I finally thought this was possible.

It is a sad and honest truth that hurts to say aloud, but I was never taught about my body: to appreciate and love the beauty of being Brown, round, and full figured. I was always too dark, too loud, too fat, too mischievous, and never feminine enough. My blatant disregard of the niceties and etiquette that young girls should perform were common reminders to my family that I was an other. And, thus, through the policing and regularization of my body through methods of whiteness, racism, and colonialism, I was taught that my body was not my own. This is an experience that is all too common for femmes who are Black, Indigenous, and People of Colour (BIPOC). And this is doubly true for those of us who are disabled. We learn that we belong to everyone but ourselves. We belong to mothers, fathers, partners, brothers, aunties, uncles, relatives we have never met, doctors, therapists, teachers, and a multitude of other figures of authority. And somehow, in this assumed ownership, these figures believe that they have earned the right to critique, mould, and shape our bodies. And because of power, privilege, and misogyny we have also been taught to let them do so, without question.

As much as I would like to forget white supremacy and racism, as I am so tired of enduring their traumas and of speaking about whiteness because it's so damn tedious, they both play/played a part in the actualization of my bodily reinvention. So naturally, it was/is through whiteness and its methods of restriction, guilt, and rage that I have come to know my body. It was only through unlearning that I came to realize that these acts of rejection were acts of colonialism—of creating borders and boundaries to make my Brownness appetizing for everyone else to consume. White supremacy and colonial beauty standards have dictated that Brown, round, and disabled femme bodies are signifiers of a difference that can only be known and actualized through the eyes of whiteness. Thus, it was/is through whiteness that I have and continue to actualize my Brown, disabled, and femme body into a reality where I can only be known through difference, through shame, and through hunger.

In many ways, I owe my life to theory. It has woken me up and given me the ability to understand the complex nature of people, politics, and social structures that govern us as human beings. But with the weight of theory, I find that another type of shame appears: the shame of vulnerability. In all honesty I have a complicated relationship with vulnerability, as I was taught that it represents weakness and, thus, an inherent flaw within a person's character. So, in being vulnerable, I must admit that I have been unable to teach myself how to love my body. This body that holds layer upon layer of a Brown magical goo of fatness that manifests as trauma and refuses to sink back into my memories. So, in writing this chapter, I choose not only resistance but resilience against the shame of vulnerability. And with this choice, I give myself permission to create a space for myself where I can embrace, write with, and express an honest vulnerability that I never thought I possessed. Going forwards with honesty and reflexivity, I must admit that with all my heart I am still fearful to publish this chapter. Quite frankly, I feel like a fraud because as I write these words down and edit them repeatedly, I cannot edit out the fact that I still have an active eating disorder. I feel ashamed of myself because despite my belief in a particular brand of politics, I am unable to translate them into action in the private spheres of my life, as a huge part of me feels unable and unwilling to let my eating disorder go. I still desire to be paper thin.

But in writing this piece and confronting my fears, I am realizing that it is okay to be in this in between space of healing—of holding on to the earthly tethers that tie my body to unrealistic ideals while simultaneously trying to let go and become wind. In saying this aloud and unpacking this heaviness my body carries, I have come to the realization that the person I have been unable to show kindness and compassion to is myself. Call it perfectionism, but I've always been too hard on myself. I have learned to beat and berate myself and not appreciate my accomplishments and hard work. Milestones have not been celebrated with joy, but instead marred with the hard determination of having only finished another task on my list. I have been consistently unable to celebrate my own successes, as I am constantly anticipating what is next. But this anticipation makes sense to me as a disabled femme of colour as my survival on it. I have not learned the lesson of how to be soft, kind, and nurturing with myself. Instead, my femme has always been a hard one—rough like the dark skin on my knees, torn and bloody, running down river with a loud exuberance.

In confronting myself and my fears, I am trying to choose a path of softness and showing my hardness a kindness that it has never known. I am choosing to hold my soft, disabled, and Brown femme body close and bathe her in the vulnerability of an honest healing that comes from the heart. To acknowledge my fears and to realize that this chapter is being written for myself and for my healing alone. I have no one to impress but myself. My soft femme truths and hard femme tears are telling me that I no longer need to feel unworthy. Instead, I should start searching inside to build a home within myself where I can feel the joy of self-love, happiness, and peace. Choosing vulnerability and honesty with the self is so difficult, but this is the journey that I have been searching for.

I have found that coming home to my femme identity is intrinsically tied to my own healing and finding the magic within myself that I have been searching for in other places. My femme continues to teach me the transformative possibilities of radical self-love as hardcore resistance mixed with a dash of sparkle and propels me into a state of new learning. About how my body can move in and through a time marked by white hetero-normative masculinities. The reclamation and reinvention of my own body has come through femme subversiveness and has taught me that this round, Brown, and disabled body of mine is mine and mine alone. My heart, mind, and soul are moving away from delegating my self-worth to the temporality of time. And each day, I am trying to challenge my beliefs that the only way to exist is through restriction, the denial of self, and my desires. By creating space for self-love, I am trying to create new memories of and for my body. But the journey of loving oneself is a daily lifelong practice that has no beginning and no ending. It instead exists on the thin line between self-compassion and kindness that occurs in the silent moments between the self and myself.

Janet Mock "believe[s] that telling our stories, first to ourselves and then to one another and the world, is a revolutionary act" (xviii). In relating Mock's wisdom to my own story, I want to begin again by telling you and me a new story, a narrative that is different from the one that I have carried for so long. My body is a story unto itself. I want to tell you and me the story of my body's incredible strength and its ability to support me through the monster of a healing journey known as long distance running. I have been running since I can remember—running away from myself, my fears, my insecurities, and my trauma. And my body still holds me up, kilometer after kilometer, despite years of emotional and physical battery fuelled by self-doubt and loathing. Long distance running has helped me to run back to myself; it has helped me to create new stories and find new ways to relate to my body, my eating disorder, and my disability. For so many years, I have been unable to trust my body. But running, just like my femme, has brought me back to myself and my centre. It has helped to create space at the sites where my body, my trauma, and self-love meet, so I can begin again and write a new story. To take baby steps on a journey that focuses on repairing the mind, body, and soul, a fracturing that began in my life so very long ago.

For years, my mother—in all her infinite wisdom and life experience—told me to start meditating. I always said "sure" with an annoyed eye roll, and I never did it. But looking back, I have been meditating since I began running as a young Brown femme—one brown foot in front of the other, step by step, and breath by breath. As each foot hits the pavement, I am reminded of how far I have come and how far I still have to go. I am reminded of how change no longer frightens me but renews me with hope. Long distance running has given me the chance to change my narrative that has been singular in its definition. It has given me the opportunity to disrupt normative conceptualizations of strength and courage via my disability and the pain my body experiences. When I run, I still experience internalized ableism and feel the physical pain of my disability. But despite the hardship that running puts my body through, the solitude of this act gives me strength to move into a place of hope. Because in the darkest and most difficult of times, hope is something you give yourself. I remember that my Brownness, my femme, and my disability are markers of my resistance and resilience. This is the hope I give myself. This is the meaning of my inner strength. Long distance running has given me hope to trust my own intuition, instead of the little voice inside of me that wants me to quit. It has become a space where I have learned that I can trust my body—to hold me, to care for me, to nurture me, and to heal me.

My body is mine, and it belongs to me. But this relationship is more than that: I belong to my body and the magic it possesses. I want this new forged relationship with my body not to have ties of ownership and possession, as those ties are wrought with practices of colonialism and patriarchy. Instead, what I want is a symbiotic relationship in which my body becomes mine, and I become my body's. I want to ask my body with kindness and tenderness to be my friend, confidante, and companion. Rooted firmly in pink granite, never swaying, and never faltering in this journey of self-love and healing. I do not own my body, and my body does not own me. Instead, what we are doing together, in conspiring with running and attuning to my disability and femmeness, is creating a type of body vulnerability that is not about judgment or shame. Instead, it is about trust and the acceptance that this road will always be a hard one. Finally, I am shedding my singular narrative and creating new stories, with each inhale and exhale on a warm spring day. Where the only company and person I need or want to be with is myself, and myself alone. I give myself permission to be infused by my own magic and to swallow this magic whole for the first time in my life. And in swallowing this magic whole, I know there is no other journey more important than this one because "when you want something, all the universe conspires in helping you to achieve it" (Coelho 23).

My body is a site of daily struggle—of race, of blood, of belonging, and never belonging. But, my body and I belong to each other. And together, each day, we are learning how to love ourselves.

Endnote

1. Femme is a queer identity. It is synonymous with queerness and hardcore resistance mixed with a dash of sparkle. Femme is not an identity that can or should be used by heterosexual people.

Works Cited

Coelho, Paulo. *The Alchemist*. Harper San Francisco, 1998.

Mock, Janet. *Redefining Realness: My Path to Womanhood, Identity, Love & So Much More.* Atria Books, 2014.

15.

the line

Tracy Royce

finally at the front of the line
you sweep your son into your ample arms
an embrace that shields his round face
from the jaundiced eye of the grocery checker
who deftly passes judgment
while scanning the canned pineapple

are you sure you wanna get him that?
she asks, pale and sylphlike
in her peach polyester smock
(her prejudice undiminished by
six years of loyal service)
one nicotine-stained finger jabbing
at your carton of ice cream
her evidence of maternal deficiency

but you hold your head high, ignore
the clucking tongues and whispers
what is she doing to that child?
eyes that read sloth and overindulgence
written on your large bodies, mistaking
dessert for a death knell, their proof
you are yet another in a long line
of women: this year's bad mommies

you could reply that your boy is strong and
healthy, and the checker's censure
would be better directed towards those
who think that flaccid celery and wilted lettuce
are good enough for working people, towards
politicians whose *ketchup is a vegetable*
ethics have harmed families far more
than ice cream ever could

but your steady gaze is reply enough
and the checker lowers her eyes
scanning the carton and mumbling
nineteen sixty-nine, please

you pay,
kiss your son,
and step away from the line.

16.

Just What the Doctor Ordered? Interrogating the Narrative of Curing the Fat Body

Kelsey Ioannoni

Having been fat for the majority of my young adult, and now adult life, making the decision to be comfortable in my fat body was not an easy one. This decision—this paradigm shift away from the dominant discourse of the thin ideal and the tyranny of slenderness (Hartley)—is the most defining feature of my life. Deciding that my health and self-worth were not intrinsically linked to my weight presented many obstacles. Overexposure to the thin ideal, dieting ads, pressure from family and friends, and, more specifically, interactions with medical professionals all act as barriers to living my bliss in my fat body.

From a young age, I have been carted around by my parents to many different medical professionals, ranging from my family doctor, paediatricians, nutritionists, therapists, psychiatrists, and more. These interactions have rarely been easy or fruitful and have often resulted in a diagnosis of obesity and a prescription for weight loss. The consequence of these appointments was a full-on war with my body. On their advice, I took many different prescription medications in effort to get control over my weight problem. For many of these drugs, weight loss was not the main purpose but an off-label result of the medication. For example, I was put on Metformin, a medication for diabetes, regardless of the fact that I am not diabetic. My doctor contended that since the off-label use of this medication was for appetite suppression and weight loss, it would be beneficial to me. Other interventions suggested by doctors were Weight Watchers, among other diet programs, and even weight loss surgery, which I applied for but did not go through with. None of these supposed so-called solutions worked in dropping pounds or obtaining a healthy or normative body mass index (BMI), and the consequences of always needing to cure my body were far reaching. I came to resent my parents and my doctors. Nothing I did seemed to work. I could not lose the weight, and, ultimately, I was never solving the weight problem. I was a failure.

My relationship with my body cannot be separated from the environment in which I came to understand weight. When I was a preteen, my sister was suffering from anorexia and spent time in hospitals and rehabilitation centres to recover. The dominant theory at the time, from my paediatrician and my family doctor, was that my weight gain was a response to my sister's rapid weight loss. Although this was never an understanding of my weight that I embraced, as a child, this theory reinforced the supposed need for medical intervention.

When I reflect back on my experiences, I put a lot of trust in my doctors to give me accurate information, and I believed what they had to say. Now, I question the authority with which many doctors prescribe weight loss as a catch-all treatment for fat people when research clearly shows that yoyo dieting and rapid weight loss lead to more negative outcomes than being fat and that the standard measures used to diagnose fat as problematic, the BMI, is flawed. In this chapter, I problematize the use of the BMI scale by medical professionals, explore conceptualizations of fatness, and conclude with an alternative perspective: Health at Every Size (HAES).

BMI: An Outdated Tool?

The BMI scale, developed over 150 years ago, is used as the primary way to measure fatness (Gard and Wright) and is calculated by dividing a person's weight in kilograms by their height squared (in metres). However, what constitutes overweight, per BMI standards, has changed throughout the years. According to Michael Gard and Jan Wright, prior to 1999, a BMI score of twenty-nine was considered overweight, which was then reduced to a BMI of twenty-seven and then to twenty-five, the current standard.

The use of the BMI scale as a measure of fatness is problematic, as, at best, BMI accounts for between 60 and 75 per cent of body fat variation in adults and is completely inaccurate for measuring body composition in children (Gard and Wright). As well, BMI fails to account for ethnic diversity or variation in body composition or the complicated relationship between weight gained and lost and health outcomes; therefore, Gard and Wright call for extreme caution in understanding statistics on obesity levels and their relation to diseases.

Criticism of the BMI scale is widespread (see, for example, Campos; Flegal et al.; Gard; Paradis). In his book *The Obesity Myth: Why America's Obsession with Weight is Hazardous to Your Health*, Paul Campos demonstrates some of the major contradictions and flaws in the medical discourses of obesity and BMI. Campos posits that the arguments for obesity as a medical problem are threefold: fat kills, thin is better for your health, and getting thin will deal with the fact that fat kills. In debunking this claim, he argues that the standard for measuring fat, BMI, is flawed. A BMI greater than twenty-five is typically claimed to be the cause of many deadly conditions, and, therefore, people need to reduce their BMI lower than twenty-five at any cost. Campos points out, however, that the negative effects of a BMI greater than twenty-five are not supported in evidence. He highlights research (for example, Waaler et al.; Ernsberger and Haskew) that demonstrates that mortality rates are actually higher in those considered underweight according to BMI.

Further research on BMI, obesity, and mortality supports the claims made by Campos and demonstrates the problematic nature of using a BMI of twenty-five as a standard. In a 2005 study conducted by Katherine Flegal et al. ("Excess Death), the researchers aimed to examine all deaths related to weight (underweight, overweight, and obesity) in the United States in 2000. The results showed an increase in mortality in both the categories of underweight (BMI <18.5) and obesity (BMI ≥ 30). The researchers found obesity to be associated with only a modest increase in relative risk of mortality. They found that overweight (BMI 25 - <30) to not be associated with any increased mortality.

In a subsequent study by Flegal et al. ("Association") in 2013, the authors found similar results and further explored this previously mentioned modest increase for those with a BMI ≥ 30. In this study,

Flegal and colleagues argue that in comparison to the normal weight category (≥18.5–<25), overweight (25–<30) is associated with significantly lower mortality rates. Flegal et al. ("Association") report that 36 per cent of adults in the United States and 24 per cent of adults in Canada have a BMI ≥ 30, making them obese. However, those who are grade one obese (BMI 30–<35) did not have significant excess mortality, which suggests that findings about the increase in excess mortality for those who are obese occur in grades two and three obesity in those with BMI ≥35.

The implications of the 2005 and 2013 studies by Flegal and her colleagues are incredible and controversial. They found in both studies that those in the category of overweight (BMI 25–<30) were at significantly lower rates of morality then those in the normal BMI range. This finding suggests that being overweight is not biomedically problematic; in fact, it appears that being overweight is healthier in terms of mortality risk than being in the normal weight category. Subsequently, their research also suggests that being grade one obese (BMI 30–<35) has no difference then the normal weight range, and the negative outcomes typically associated with those who are grade two or three obese are not that straightforward either. The BMI scale is used as a standard in measuring a healthy weight; however, this research, which is a review of much of the existing research on weight and mortality, shows that the negative health consequences in relation to mortality do not occur for at least ten points higher on the BMI scale than what is used as the cap for what is considered normal body weight (BMI <25). This begs the question: Why do we continue to use the BMI scale as a standard? Indeed, BMI exists as an ever-shrinking standard, as the change in the construction of the normal category of BMI has been shrinking since 1999.

The BMI scale has always been a source of frustration in understanding my personal health. I cannot count the number of times ever since I was a preteen that I have been shown the BMI chart, whereby my height and weight always place me in the obese zone. My doctor would take out the laminated chart, point to my height. and point out where my healthy weight should fall. This ranged from about 120 to 135 pounds, as I grew in height. She would then ominously point out where, in fact, my weight was on the chart—always in the obese or extremely obese section.

As an adult, I have relinquished the powerful hold that BMI held on me. As a teenager, however, BMI and the BMI chart haunted me. My BMI held a torturous grip on my conceptualizations of my health. In my preteen, early teenage years, I was about five foot one. To have a healthy BMI, or as my doctor would tell me, to be healthy, I would need to be a maximum of about 125 pounds, but I should aim to be about between 110 and 115 pounds. At the time, I was closer to, if not already, two hundred pounds, with a BMI of thirty nine and bordering on extremely obese. I was a failure.

Health, Fatness, and the Doctor

In her work "Doctor's Orders: Diagnosis, Medical Authority, and the Exploitation of the Fat Body," Annemarie Jutel explores the pathologization of weight and how there exists an assumption that body size is indicative of individual nature. She links this relationship with beauty and argues that the link between health and beauty is historical. As Jutel indicates that cultural values influence the fluidity of classifying conditions as disease, she argues that these values around health and beauty have seeped into medical practice, influencing the categorization of overweight as a disease.

Jutel points out that there exists a circular relationship between health and anxiety. The diagnosis of overweight reflects societal belief in the relationship between health and appearance. At the same time, however, the power of medicine as an institution uses science to validate the anxieties of the public and reinforce the power of medicine in social control. Jutel argues that the reproduction of anxieties and the diagnostic process through the power of medicine contribute to the exploitation of overweight people, as the medicalization of weight opens up commercial interests and industries that benefit from the classification of overweight as a disease.

In *Fat Genes and the Obesity Blame Game,* Eric Oliver discusses the set point theory of homeostasis, which means that people maintain a balance between weight and energy. The set point of weight, Oliver argues, is why people see little success with dieting. As people lose weight while dieting, the body tries to compensate for the lost weight by, for example, retaining more water, in attempts to regain homeostasis. According to Oliver, "The set point theory of weight suggests that substantial and sustained weight loss is going to be nearly impossible for anyone with a high weight range" (108).

The obesity epidemic is one of the most powerful discourses that influences the way in which health and bodies are conceptualized. Jan Wright argues that the alleged truths about the obesity epidemic have been reconceptualized by government policy, health promotion initiatives, online resources, and in-school practices that influence the way in which young people come to understand themselves. Children and young people come to know themselves in ways that have been constructed by claims makers.

The pathologization of my weight is how I came to know my body as a young person. I grew up understanding my body as a site of contestation and a site of failure—a body in need of a cure. This understanding of my body as a failure and as in need of change permeated my life. I felt as though I was living on a battlefield, my brain a soldier against its enemy, my fat flesh, and this was not a war I was going to win. Throughout my teenage years, my parents and my doctors would question whether I was actually putting the effort in to lose the weight, as they frequently told me weight loss should be as simple as calories in versus calories out. The contestant questioning, masked as concern, felt laced with accusations that I was not working hard enough and that I did not care about the impact of my weight on my health.

The barrage of messaging around weight loss, coming from those who care the most about me, created a contentious relationship between myself, my body, and food. Disordered eating practices and thought patterns around food were not something I was unfamiliar with; at the same time that my parents were seeking help about my obesity, my sister was being treated for severe anorexia. Yet the disordered practices that were being corrected with her—behaviours like severe caloric restrictions, calorie counting, excessive exercise, and obsessive thinking about weight—were being prescribed to me in order to foster weight loss. The same behaviours being corrected in my thin, sick sister were being instilled in me as a fat child. It was not until I was in my early twenties that I learned that there are healthier relationships I could have with my body—relationships that do not result in self-hatred, shame, and feelings of failure but, in fact, accept and celebrate my fatness.

Reconceptualizing Health: Health at Every Size

Current understandings of fatness are constructed through our historical, cultural, and economic positions (LeBesco), and fat activists have been challenging the marginalized understandings of fatness for over forty years. As such, there has been a radical r-imagination of fatness and health called "health at every size" (HAES) (see Bacon and Aphramor, Bacon et al., and Burgard).

Research on the supposed success of dieting as a method of weight loss has been heavily criticized (see Campos; Oliver; LeBesco; Gailey; and Lyons). Linda Bacon et al. have noted how dieting is a new part of our cultural identity, and this creates many problems, as the effects of dieting can have negative impacts on people's bodies (Lyons). Instead, they call for rethinking conceptualizations of health, a shift to an understanding of health that focuses on intuitive eating that relies on body cues, and the promotion of a model of health that does not equate health with size.

The HAES perspective focuses on living a healthy life through healthy practices, which include positive self-acceptance. The HAES model challenges the use of the BMI scale in understanding what is a healthy body. According to Deb Burgard, health is "the process of daily life rather than the outcome of weight" (43).

Clinical studies, such as ones conducted by Bacon et al., that compare HAES with forms of weight loss treatment found that HAES has sustained health improvements across many indicators of health, such as psychological and physiological measures. HAES is shown to significantly effect healthy living practices in the long term (Bacon et al)

In her research on BMI as a normative discourse, Christine Halse argues that the BMI norm "has progressively colonized the policies, practices, and procedures for measuring and documenting weight" (46). Normative BMI as a virtue discourse is moralistic and reinforces the thin ideal rooted in a culture of thinness. Constructing BMI as a normative understanding of weight and its supposed relationship to a myriad of health problems results in people reinforcing this discourse by regulating themselves.

In contrast, the HAES model embraces diversity in body size and weight and recognizes the importance of understanding health as practice, not as weight. HAES challenges the normative discourse perpetuated by BMI-driven health practices (see Bacon and Aphramor,

Bacon et al., and Burgard). The disentanglement of weight and BMI from health has been transformative in my life.

I have had little to no success as a dieter, and the resulting discouragement further influenced my interest in engaging in health practices, as these practices never bore out the ultimate goal of weight loss. Accepting my body as fat and living happily in the body I have versus the body society thinks I should have were the healthiest decisions I have ever made for myself. No longer do I anguish over having a specific BMI that has arbitrarily been designated as healthy, nor do I focus on weight loss as defining my goal of healthy living. Instead, I see health as practice, and shifting to understanding myself in a HAES framework has allowed me to appreciate myself in ways I have not before.

My relationship with my body is a journey, and my paradigm shift is fairly recent. But as I dip my toes into the waters of HAES and explore the literature available, both academically and socially, on fatness, I have let go of my hatred for my body. Instead, I embrace myself as a fat woman and work hard to enjoy my life as it is. My fatness no longer stands in the way of my happiness.

Works Cited

Bacon, Linda, and Lucy Aphramor. "Weight Science: Evaluating the Evidence for a Paradigm Shift." *Nutrition Journal*, vol. 10, no. 9, 2011, pp. 1-14.

Bacon, Linda, et al. "Size Acceptance and Intuitive Eating Improve Health for Obese, Female Chronic Dieters." *Journal of the American Dietetic Association*, vol. 105, no. 6, 2005, pp. 929-36.

Burgard, Deb. "What is Health at Every Size?" *The Fat Studies Reader*, edited by Esther Rothblum and Sondra Solovay, New York University Press, 2009, pp. 41-53.

Campos, Paul. *The Obesity Myth: Why America's Obsession with Weight is Hazardous To Your Health.* Gotham, 2004.

Ernsberger, Paul, and Paul Haskew. "Health Implications of Obesity: An Alternative View." *Journal of Obesity and Weight Regulation*, vol. 6, 1987, p. 67.

Flegal, Katherine, et al. "Excess Death Associated with Underweight and Obesity." *Journal of American Medical Association* 293.15 (2005): 1861-67.

Flegal, Katherine, et al. "Association of All-Cause Mortality with Overweight and Obesity Using Standard Body Mass Index Categories." *Journal of American Medical Association*, vol. 309, no. 1, 2013, pp. 71-82.

Gailey, Jeannine. *The Hyper(in)visible Fat Woman*. Palgrave Macmillan, 2014.

Gard, Michael, and Jan Wright. *The Obesity Epidemic: Science, Morality and Ideology*. Taylor & Francis Inc, 2005.

Gard, Michael. "Hearing Noises and Noticing Silence: Towards A Critical Engagement With Canadian Body Weight Statistics." *Obesity in Canada: Critical Perspectives*, edited by Jenny Ellison, Deborah McPhail, and Wendy Mitchinson, University of Toronto Press, 2016, pp. 31-55.

Halse, Christine. "Biocitizenship: Virtue Discourses and the Birth of the Biocitizen." *Biopolitics and the "Obesity Epidemic": Governing Bodies*, edited by Jan Wright and Valerie Harwood, Routledge, 2009, pp. 44-59.

Hartley, Cecilia. "Letting Ourselves Go: Making Room for the Fat Body in Feminist Scholarship." *Bodies out of Bounds: Fatness and Transgression*, edited by Jana Evans Braziel and Kathleen LeBesco, University of California Press, 2001, pp. 245-54.

Jutel, Annemarie. "Doctor's Orders: Diagnosis, Medical Authority and the Exploitation of the Fat Body." *Biopolitics and the "Obesity Epidemic": Governing Bodies*, edited by Jan Wright and Valerie Harwood, Routledge, 2009, pp. 60-77.

LeBesco, Kathleen. *Revolting Bodies? The Struggle to Redefine Fat Identity*. University of Massachusetts Press, 2004.

Lyons, Pat. "Prescription for Harm: Diet Industry Influence, Public Health Policy, and the 'Obesity Epidemic.'" *The Fat Studies Reader*, edited by Esther Rothblum and Sondra Solovay, New York University Press, 2009, pp. 75-87.

Oliver Eric. *Fat Politics: The Real Story Behind America's Obesity Epidemic*. Oxford University Press, 2005.

Paradis, Elise. "'Obesity' as Process: The Medicalization of Fatness by Canadian Researchers, 1971-2010." *Obesity in Canada: Critical Perspectives*, edited by Jenny Ellison, Deborah McPhail, and Wendy Mitchinson, University of Toronto, 2016, pp. 56-88.

Waaler, Hans. "Height, Weight, and Mortality: The Norwegian Experience." *Acta Medica Scandinavia*, vol. 679, 1987, pp. 1-56.

Wright, Jan. "Biopower, Biopedagogies, and the Obesity Epidemic." *Biopolitics and the "Obesity Epidemic": Governing Bodies*, edited by J. Wright and V. Harwood, Routledge, 2009, pp. 1-14.

17.

Body Lessons

Sonja Boon

Seventy-five kilograms. That's what the scale says. That dusty yellow one that lives under the bathroom cabinet. It only reads in kilograms. And it says seventy-five. Your father records this in the calendar you got for free from the Re/Max realtor, the one that hangs in the kitchen and lists all the important dates and information. Last week, it said seventy-four. Last month, it said seventy-three. You know your mother's friends will see it.

Your mother registers you for aerobics. It's a special class, just for teens.

"It will be good for you," she says. You hear, "You're too fat" because that's what she really means. When you come home from school, there are diet books on your bed, strategically placed at an angle, near the foot, on top of the granny square bedspread crocheted by a grandmother with arthritic fingers so stiff that she couldn't even bend them anymore. In the kitchen there are yogurt tubs filled with carrot sticks and celery sticks. Your mother cuts them up on the weekend and soaks them in cold water so they'll stay fresh, but all that happens is that they start to bend and curl. Misshapen stalks reminding you that you are misshapen, too. In the summer, she'll register you for the swim team. No is not an option.

Teen aerobics is at the Legion Hall, where city councillors make pancakes on Canada Day and where, when you are seventeen, you will start going to donate blood. But you're getting ahead of yourself because right now you are sixteen, and here you are—look at you—lying on a mat on the shiny, waxed floor of the multipurpose room trying to hear your instructor over the pounding music.

Curl your legs in. Hold for four. 1, 2, 3, 4. Watch your tummy!

Ernie's mom teaches aerobics. Maybe her name is Cathy. You can't remember. But you've known Ernie since grade two at least because that's when you became his hands after he fell off the garage roof and broke both his arms. Or was it when he burned himself after playing with matches? You're not sure. But this much is true: You wrote his assignments for six weeks, and you didn't even get behind because you were already so far ahead. Ernie has a little brother, you seem to recall, but you can't remember his name. and really, for this story, Ernie's brother and his arms and what exactly happened to them don't really matter. What matters is Ernie's mom. She's tiny and trim with frizzy, overpermed hair.

Turn on your side. Pump those legs up. And one, and two, and three, and four.

Ernie's mom is perky in her bodysuit with leg warmers. Don't laugh. You're in the *Flashdance* years, and you wanted leg warmers too, more than anything, but you didn't get the fancy fuzzy cream and brown ones that the popular girls wear. This class, it bears noting, is all popular girls. Except for you, that is. Your leg warmers came from the Army and Navy store in Edmonton where the only remotely tolerable colour was grey, and so that's what you bought. But when you put them over your jeans, you realized that they weren't remotely tolerable at all and decided to abandon all pretense of fashion.

March in place. Heads up. Smile! And one, two, three, four. Push those knees right up to your chest!

And here you are, with all the popular girls with their long, curled hair and bangs teased right to the sky. Hairspray. You can smell it when they walk past. They all have Braun curling irons, those white ones with black wands that fit right into your purse, cuddling up next to the hairspray. You have a curling iron, too. But it's from Canadian Tire. It's big, brown, and bulky.

Kick your legs forwards and back and forwards and back. And now your arms. Clap forwards. Clap back. Forwards. Back.

The popular girls have perfect makeup and perfect bodysuits and perfect popular girl leg warmers. They smile at you, perfect smiles, but they'll ignore you at school. You despise them. But you've been raised to be polite.

Lunge left. Lunge right. Left and right. Now forwards and back. Forwards and back. Push it. Pump it. One, two, three, four.

Look at you in your baby pink sweats. Zellers this time, Londonderry Mall. And here's another reason you need to remind people that you've abandoned all pretense. Because then you can say you meant it. Remember, you're the one telling the story, and you need to tell it your way.

And so, in your story, you're a rebel. Own that title. Speak that truth, sister. Deep inside, you know the real story. You're a fighter, but you're too scared to show it. You speak out. You speak back. You're sassy. You kick ass. You really do. But it's all in your head. Because on the outside, pink lady, you're soft, meek, and pliant. You do what you need to do, and you don't say much. Everything you say can and will be used against you. That much you've learned.

Arms up. Breathe in. Arms down. Breathe out. That's it. Let your body relax.

When you're finally pretzeled into a modified lotus position, Ernie's mom tells you that the camera makes you look ten pounds heavier. Or more. It could be fifteen, but you can't quite remember. The problem is that you need to translate this back into kilograms. What will the yellow scale say?

And all of this runs through your brain, years later, when you are in the middle of playing the *Rondo* from Mozart's *Quartet in D major* on Canada AM just before your chamber music tour to Japan. You've got your skinny skirt on, but it's entirely possible that you still look fat, and if your mother is watching you know she'll have noticed.

"She looks fat," she'll say to your father, echoing your thoughts. And he'll nod in that distracted, absent-minded way and go back to his work.

Suggested Readings

Bordo, Susan. *Unbearable Weight: Feminism, Western Culture, and the Body.* University of California Press, 2004.

Ellingson, Laura L. "Embodied Knowledge: Writing Researchers' Bodies into Qualitative Health Research." *Qualitative Health Research*, vol. 16, no. 2, 2006, pp. 298-310.

Farrell, Amy Erdman. *Fat Shame: Stigma and the Fat Body in American Culture.* New York University Press, 2011.

Grosz, Elizabeth. *Volatile Bodies: Toward a Corporeal Feminism*. Indiana University Press, 1994.

Hartley, Cecelia. "Letting Ourselves Go: Making Room for the Fat Body in Feminist Scholarship." *Bodies Out of Bounds: Fatness and Transgression*, edited by Jane Evans Braziel and Kathleen LeBesco, University of California Press, 2001, pp. 60-73.

LeBesco, Kathleen. "Queering Fat Bodies/Politics." *Bodies Out of Bounds: Fatness and Transgression*, edited by Jane Evans Braziel and Kathleen LeBesco, University of California Press, 2001, pp. 74-87.

LeBesco, Kathleen. *Revolting Bodies: The Struggle to Redefine Fat Identity*. University of Massachusetts Press, 2004.

Murray, Samantha. "Corporeal Knowledges and Deviant Bodies: Perceiving the Fat Body." *Social Semiotics*, vol. 17, no. 3, 2007, pp. 361-73.

Murray, Samantha. "(Un/Be)Coming Out? Rethinking Fat Politics." *Social Semiotics*, vol. 15, no. 2, 2005, pp. 153-63.

Rice, Carla. "Becoming the "Fat Girl": Acquisition of an Unfit Identity." *Women's Studies International Forum*, vol. 30, no. 2, 2007, pp. 158-74.

Rice, Carla. *Becoming Women: The Embodied Self in Image Culture*. University of Toronto Press, 2014.

Wann, Marilyn. *Fat!So?* Ten Speed Press, 1998.

18.

"Here Comes Fat May": Learning and Relearning to Love My Body

May Lui

Family

It always starts with family doesn't it? My Chinese father and my Jewish mother met in the early 1960s and married in 1962 in Montréal, Québec, Canada. I was born in 1966, a middle child in a mixed-race family.

Loving my fat body has been an ongoing lifelong learning journey for me. It's been a struggle, a war, with some acceptance, bursts of love. Repeat. My personal story is a kaleidoscope of shared pieces, thoughts, and moments in time woven imperfectly together.

"Here comes Fat May!"

This was my father's greeting to me in the mornings when I was a teenager, coming downstairs for breakfast. I hated when he spoke to me that way; his calm or laughing words were like casually tossed jagged rocks at my tender heart. Decades later, my Chinese friends would tell me that being from China, he had learned this as a common way for Chinese parents to speak to children. Although I reject this, since as an adult I've met many Chinese parents that don't do this, as a teen without any Chinese friends, I had no cultural references. Sometimes, he'd narrate: "Fat May is making toast! Fat May is getting orange juice!"

My mother would say, "If you just lost a bit of weight, you'd look so nice." She'd gently touch me on the side of my face. "You'd be so lovely," she'd say wistfully, her words slicing my ego, heart, and self. In more frustrating moments, she'd raise her voice and say, "Stop eating so much! Do you want to be as big as a house?"

Food

In my mixed cultural upbringing in the suburban and urban metropolises of Montreal and Toronto, food was more than food. For my Jewish mother and her family, food is love, comfort, and nurturing. Food is what we talk about when we don't want to talk about real things. For my Chinese father, food was celebration, family, duty, and togetherness. I remember the merged foods of the everyday: congee, brisket, latkes, chasew, smoked meat sandwiches with rye bread and caraway seeds, Montreal bagels (vive le St. Viateur!), har gow, and ho fun noodles. I love food. I love eating with friends and original, chosen, and found family. Pesach, lunar new year, Jewish brunches, dim sum weekends. Eat, eat!

Food also comforts other hungers. Food is more than food. It connects me to my culture and heritage. It also soothes hurt, sadness, and loneliness, as well as anger and frustration.

School

I loved music. Starting from age six, I took piano lessons. I started playing the cello in middle school at age eleven and continued into high school. I loved when I practiced on my own but especially loved making music with others. Playing in an orchestra taught me to listen to others, and I was thrilled by the music we all made together. I felt grounded in my body playing the cello, holding it to me, feeling the instrument and feeling pride and happiness with how my skills grew.

I also loved singing and joined choirs in high school and continue to sing with gusto when I'm alone. And I loved math and logic. I loved reading and writing. I wrote bad poetry. I read everything written by Judy Blume, Beverly Cleary, and Laura Ingles Wilder. I imagined myself in the all-white families of the stories I read—thin and white, with all my problems resolved by the end of the book.

Body Theory, Body Real

In 1986, at age nineteen, I moved out. I had part-time jobs and went to university part time. I discovered feminism, reclaimed my mixed-race identity, and found antiracism, anticolonialism, socialism, and queer theory. I learned many empowering ideas, practices, and actions.

I loved finding writers who had been writing about these realities for years, finally putting words and language to ideas and thoughts I'd had for so long: bell hooks. Himani Bannerji. Noam Chomsky. I became an activist, went to rallies, marches. I yelled in the streets. I was always interested in many causes, such as Against Cruise Testing,[1] International Women's Day, Take Back the Night, and Ontario Days of Action. After I came out, I went to Pride marches and Dyke marches. I found a way to externalize my feelings of being powerless against huge forces by making small moments of change bit by bit. Being united with others in sameness and difference, even for those fleeting moments in the streets, moved and empowered me in ways words never could.

Even more shifted for me as I found the feminist critique of the female beauty ideal. Naomi Wolf's *The Beauty Myth* was revolutionary to me at the time. (The critiques would come later.) I learned about the multi-million (at the time, now in the billions) dollar weight-loss industry. I read the most radical words I'd ever read to that point: What if women stopped hating our bodies? What if women stopped spending money trying to lose weight, trying to attain an unattainable beauty ideal? What if we took that energy and turned it into something positive? What would happen? Many industries would simply collapse and fold in on themselves, as worthless and useless as they've always been, without us holding up their flawed ideology, always holding happiness out of reach of the fat girls.

And beyond beauty ideals—which are simply not attainable for many of us based on racist, classist, heteronormative, cis-centric, and ableist notions of beauty—what about the complexity of the idea of beauty? What about the multifaceted world that is women, femmes, and femme-identified trans and queer folks? Aren't we more than what we look like?

I began to understand the imperialist functions of racist, homophobic, and classist social constructions of beauty, and I reimagined women's body image under a critical feminist, anti-racist, anti-colonial lens. Kill the cop in your head. Fuck your racist beauty standards!

In the 1990s Ms. Magazine had a feature called "No Comment," in which blatantly sexist ads were shown, with no comments added or needed. In 1998, I read Fat?So! by Marilyn Wann. In 1999, Fireweed Feminist Quarterly published their fat issue. In 2000, I read Camryn Manheim's memoir Wake Up I'm Fat! I read these texts like the precious gems they were, speaking of a reality in which I wished to literally embody myself, wrapping myself with words of empowerment, wishing I could absorb them like water. Around the same time, I saw Margaret Cho's comeback solo show I'm the One That I Want and loved her for taking up space, being loud, being Asian, swearing on stage, being a queer-positive feminist, and wearing a tight outfit with her rolls showing. I wished I could be like her.

And yet.

I'd look in the mirror or catch a glimpse of myself in a storefront window in downtown Toronto on College Street or Bloor Street and think, "*Wow she's fat! Who is that disgusting person? How can people even stand to look at me? I can't.*"

I was and am more abusive to myself than any yelled taunt, whispered tease, or a "Here comes Fat May!"

I didn't believe the theory. Despite learning more, reading empowering texts, even as I said it to others, I didn't always believe it.

Sometimes, I think that if I say it often enough, I'll believe it. That works. Sometimes, I think that if I surround myself with friends who love their bodies, who talk about fat shaming in critical feminist ways, this will help. It does. I like to talk about body positivity as a journey, not a destination. That works too.

Patriarchal, racist, classist, homophobic, ableist, and colonial Canadian society tells me, and all women, that what we look like matters more than anything else about us. It also tells us we will never be pretty enough, never be light enough, never be skinny enough, and never be attractive enough.

I try to interrupt the negative voice, change the topic like an uncomfortable conversation with family, and decide to think about positive ways that I love my body. Then slowly, over time, with lots of ups and downs, I can do something different, something more positive, something that actually makes me happy. It takes time, patience and care, characteristics I share effortlessly with friends, lovers, family, and others but far less so with myself. Learning and relearning to love my body is, like any practice, ongoing; it involves creating more muscle memory or heart memory and making a conscious decision to ignore the voice that has never brought me joy or pleasure.

Sex

I had my first lover at the age of nineteen. After a year of dating, we moved in together and lived together for three years. I had lots of firsts, my first real date, my first "butterflies in the stomach" feeling, my first time having sex, my first orgasm, and my first time living away from my parents. And the first time I had good sex. What's good sex? At the time, it was connected with love, trust, openness, and a vulnerability I hadn't known before. Not only was I a virgin, I was also completely sexually inexperienced. Sex for me was connected with love. Being naked was never something I felt comfortable with, but I could escape the idea of being naked in the dark and semidark. Good sex felt like letting go, feeling the point of no return wash over like a hard, pounding, throbbing, shaking wave of freedom in my body in a wonderful, delicious way.

But how I felt about my body didn't change. I didn't really think that he was attracted to me or that he enjoyed my body or that he was aroused by my body, even though there was much evidence that he did and was. I'm not sure what I thought about his attraction for me. His attention and how good sex felt still didn't dislodge my hatred of my body.

In the waning year of our relationship (early 1990s), I read Adrienne Rich's "Compulsory Heterosexuality." My mind was officially blown. What? Being straight was taught and not natural? I could be attracted to women? Was I attracted to women? Spoiler alert: Yes, I was.

Queerness

A few years later, in my mid-twenties, while working in frontline social services, I developed a crush on a lesbian coworker. I called myself straight, with a crush on a woman. I insisted this was true. My colleagues and friends smiled at me and waited. It wasn't long before I came out.

I started noticing women's bodies, all women's bodies, but especially large women. In the mid-to-late 1990s when I was in my early thirties and in graduate school, I became friends with a large woman who wore tank tops, not seeming to care about her large upper arms, a part of my body that I really don't like. I was amazed by her lack of self-consciousness and began to wear tank tops myself, struggling to feel comfortable with my upper arms. Around the same time, a friend introduced me to the musical group Sweet Honey in the Rock, and I was astounded by the clothes the women wore. They were large Black women. They wore bright colours! Patterns! They were beautiful. I began to search for more than just baggy tops, solids, and darker colours to keep me invisible. I began to search for visibility.

As far as actual sex, there were a few awkward dates, some fumbling sexual attempts (and failures), many unrequited crushes, and one hot encounter at a women's bathhouse evening, making out with a group of six or seven women. It was a moment filled with momentary exhilaration, fun, acceptance, and lust.

Walking along city streets today, I see young Asian and white women, fat and proud, with bright pink, purple, and green hair, wearing stripes and tight leggings and cropped tops with their belly rolls showing, wearing tops with no sleeves. I read them as queer, since isn't it queer and radical and extraordinary to be fat and colourful in this world that hates us? They show their arms, their bellies, and their lovely thick thighs in public with pleasure and love. I smile at them. I am happy they exist in the world.

Sex, Again

In 2003, in my mid-thirties, I had my second serious relationship. After many years identifying as lesbian, I shifted toward identifying as bisexual. Hearing other women talk about their bodies, including women who were, what I term, attractive-by-society's-standards, shifted me. I suppose this lover arrived at a time when I could receive what he had to give. He was very sexual. He loved and lusted after my body. I was able to hear his touches, feel the loving intent, and taste and absorb sex in ways I hadn't before.

I was published in a sex anthology, *With a Rough Tongue: Femmes Write Porn*. My piece was called "Yes Means Yes." My first and only published erotica writing. The lusty lover who changed my life, my partner at the time, came with me to some of the book launches. I remember the big launch at Buddies in Bad Times in Toronto. I wore a red dress, tight and clingy, and we arrived at the venue early. He had brought his fancy camera and asked me to get on the empty stage so he could snap photos of me. "No!" I said, automatically rejecting my body being the focus of attention. "Why would you want to do that?" I asked. He lovingly insisted, so I stepped up and felt a surge of love, kindness, acceptance, and the realness of his feelings. He wants to take photos of me. He really does. It was unreal to know this was true.

Because of this lover, I discovered my kinky side. I discovered more ways, kinds, and intensities of pleasure and orgasm, and ways that my body gave me and my subsequent lovers pleasure. It was, and continues to be, an astounding gift that I value and cherish.

From him, I learned that validation is good when it comes from within, but sometimes external forces can give it a good solid push.

Dragonboat

I joined an amateur dragonboat team in 2014—the Rusty Dragon Adventures, Harbord Village team. I'm a bit creaky sometimes, in my knees, but it was an amateur neighbourhood league that required no particular level of fitness. Perfect! The first few practices, that first year when I had no idea what I was doing, were incredible. I loved learning the dragonboat paddle stroke, being on the water, communing with the waterfowl during breaks, and being part of a team. I learned that we move faster if we are all paddling together. How ironic that I had eschewed team sports and competition for most of my life. Today, dragonboat racing has become a wonderful new practice for me, and the competitions, while a small part of the process, actually push me to achieve more. I love it. The season is short, May to late September or early October, and I savour the practices in the calm bays of Lake Ontario, getting splashed every so often, laughing and loving the sport. I love how I feel in my body when I've completed a good practice.

The (Ongoing) End

Today, I can say that while there is always more work to be done, I have internalized and absorbed theory. I see and appreciate beautiful, large, and rounded women. I have many amazing orgasms. I more and more feel that my body is beautiful and that I am beautiful the way I am. There is less and less separation of my body and me.

Turning fifty allowed me to reflect on my friends, who I've loved and who I love now. I reflect on how they provide me strength, support, and love in my life. I'm more than my body, but I'm also so grateful for all that my body has survived with me.

I still catch glimpses of myself in storefront windows. I now smile at myself and say "Hey, I'm cute!" or "Wow my butt looks good today!" The voice is more silent than it's ever been and gets more silent with each victory I live. And I move forwards, smiling a soft smile out to the world.

Endnote

1. Against Cruise Testing was a social movement in the 1980s as activists in England, Canada, and the United States protested the emergence of cruise missiles, which are guided high-speed missiles with large warheads.

Acknowledgments

Thanks to my friends who have supported me along the way: Anjula Gogia for your friendship for all those years at Toronto Women's Bookstore; Penney Kirby for decades of friendship and so many talks about family, fatness, and food; Helen Luu for introducing me to dragonboating; and Jill Andrew for being beautiful, affirming, fun, and so smart.

19.

My New Skin–Tattoos and Skin-Deep Body Love

Dorothée Jankuhn

(Warning: This chapter includes content about body dysmorphic disorder, dissociative behavior, and eating disorders.)

Let me tell you about my new skin and what she is doing for me every day. I grew up hating my body. I know that a lot of womxn experience this, but for me personally, it didn't just stop at body dissatisfaction; it went straight to body dysmorphic disorder. By that, I specifically mean I was disgusted when I looked at myself in the mirror, let alone when I felt my body. The squish of my fat, the roundness of my hips, my short legs, and my round belly with its big rolls—I deemed all that unattractive and, therefore, disgusting. This wouldn't stop with the end of puberty; it kept on going, but no one was really interested in hearing a fat girl complain, so I kept my thoughts to myself. In order to cope, I slowly began to think of my body and my mind as two separate entities. Because I did not want to acknowledge my body anymore, I deliberately broke off connection to it. I was asking myself "How can my beautiful mind live in something so repulsive?"

My journey towards body love began after I met my primary partner. He helped me reestablish a connection to my body. For the first time in years, I was finally able to see her[1] as part of me, as connected to my mind, instead of an annoying shell, which I reluctantly had to take care of.

I was in the process of moving towards a practice of body truce when suddenly and unexpectedly my mother passed away. After the initial shock, I developed an eating disorder, resulting in me putting on a considerable amount of weight in a short period of time. Even though this might seem like a setback, my first thoughts were not about the weight but about how I ate. I quickly realized that my eating patterns weren't normal, and they didn't feel right to me; it felt like a forced behaviour in order to be able to cope with my loss. I decided to seek help. After searching the internet and local libraries for anything about my eating disorder trying to understand what happened to me, I stumbled upon body positivity and eventually fat acceptance. One radical question stuck inside my head: "What if it were okay to be fat?" My initial reaction was disbelief, but over time, it marinated in my head the more I would read about fat activism, body liberation, and breaking away from toxic diet culture.

It felt like I was getting sucked into a whirlwind of information and empowerment from that moment on. Of course, accepting my body didn't happen overnight. It was a long and rocky road, but finally I had more good body days than bad body days, and that was a first for me.

It was then that I felt the need to get my second tattoo done, to literally inscribe this personal success into my skin. My family had a love of fairytales, and I was lucky to grow up with all sorts of myths and stories. Among them were the tales of Baron of Münchhausen. The story of Münchhausen accidentally riding his horse into a swamp and saving himself from drowning by pulling himself out by his own hair stuck with me. I didn't understand the deeper psychological and philosophical meaning of this picture as a child of course. Only after accomplishing something I never deemed possible did I remember this tale, and I could feel something inside me just falling into place when thinking of this image. However, I did not want a picture of a man on his horse in full feudal uniform in my skin. Almost instantly—the story of Lady Godiva, a noblewoman who bravely rode her horse across town naked in order to help the people of Coventry in the United Kingdom—came to my mind. I quickly decided to mash up the two tales and have a Lady Godiva who pulls herself out of the swamp by her own hair on and inside my skin.

My first tattoo-related body love moment was when the artist first put the stencil of the design on me to check the placement. I looked at my thigh in the mirror and immediately started to jiggle it and fell in love with how the design moved when I moved. It almost looked as if a part of the design was jumping joyfully, which instantly made me love my thigh even more. So much so, that to this day I have never wished for thinner thighs or a thigh gap.

Getting a larger tattoo is different from getting one that can be done in half an hour, like my first one. I had to go to the tattoo studio for several sessions and commit to a cycle of getting painfully tattooed, healing, and the returning for the next session. After each session, I would leave with a medical membrane attached to my skin, which was put on the fresh wound to shield it from dirt, which had to be removed after two days. To me, this felt like shedding my old skin, like snakes do. It was an intensely liberating practice for me, almost like renewing myself after every single session. While carefully pulling off the membrane, I imagined getting rid of all the hurtful micro- and in-my-face aggressions or fatphobic bullying in general that I had received in my life. I could feel that I was leaving an old part of myself behind for something new. The whole tattoo aftercare process felt like a ritual to me as well. After the shedding of the old skin, came the ritual washing (cleaning of the excess ink, blood, and goo under the membrane). After that, there was ritual embalming, which meant using special tattoo ointment to help the skin heal. But all ritual allegories aside, taking care of my new skin turned out to be a delicate business. After an episode of bad healing, I found out that there is no universal tattoo aftercare routine, and I was the only one responsible for taking good care of my new skin and determining what and how much I would do to ensure good healing. I had to listen to her needs. Skin is alive, so there were parts of the tattoo that were dryer than others and needed a little extra care and attention. I had to also apply ointment every other day but not too much and not too little. Improper care would wash out the ink or cause skin irritations. This was a no brainer. During the whole aftercare process, I absolutely had to touch my body more frequently than I would normally. One of the most interesting parts was that I started talking to my tattoo, and this actually felt really nice. While inspecting it regularly for dry parts, I would ask, "How are you today? Do you need some extra care somewhere? What can I do for you to feel better?" Questions I honestly would ask myself only scarcely. I wondered why I was not talking to my whole body benevolently like that more often. I made the deliberate decision to do so. After every other shower, bath, or whenever I feel the need to do so, I now take the time to put deliciously smelling body lotion on my whole body and massage it in gently while telling her, "I love you just the way you are, and I'm sorry for all the years I treated you so poorly. You deserve to be treated with respect! You are a part of me. You are brave and incredibly strong because you survived all the awful stuff that happened to you—the diets I put you through, the neglect, the bullying, and the exercise you didn't like. You survived all of this, and I promise to take better care of you and listen to your needs."

Although I got my tattoo to celebrate my newfound body positivity, the tattoo has done so much more for me. It helped me to establish a new meaningful relationship with my skin and my whole body by putting art on a big part of my skin, which is not only beautiful to me but also reminds me of my journey to self-acceptance and ultimately self-love. I definitely no longer feel disgusted when I look at my body in the mirror anymore. Weirdly, I also feel less naked because I have the feeling of always wearing something beautiful if that makes sense. Even on a bad body day, I look at my thigh and I'm reminded that I have overcome tough moments in my life. I managed to heal my relationship with food and my body, and I'm working on healing past traumas one step at a time. I finally am able to see myself through loving, benevolent eyes like my partner sees me. Not just my tattoo, my whole body is a beautiful work of art and deserves the same love and respect. By making the conscious decision to commemorate my success with something that will last, my tattoo acts as a constant reminder, a touchstone if you will, of my pulling myself out of the metaphorical swamp of body hatred, body shame, internalized fatphobia, as well as grief for my mother. It is important for me to stress this because as a person suffering from depression, I need to be able to see my accomplishments in an undeniable way when my depression is getting a hold of me again. With my tattoo, I am telling my personal body love story—my ongoing quest for peace and healing in my own skin. I am showing empowerment and agency because I chose it for myself.

Endnotes

1. I identify my body as female; therefore, I use the pronouns she and her.

20.

A Call for Self-Love

Tierra Hohn

My body is my temple
Yet I have constantly deceived it
If that dress did not fit, then my answer was "NO"; no I am not eating it

Views, distorted
Vision, blurred
But what I have realized, now, is that society's standards are absurd
I cannot fit that "ideal" model
There is no standard human being
We are unique creatures
All beautiful with individual meaning

My body is the instrument
That brings to life the inhibitions of my mind
Though, society demands that my body be confined
To the measurements and expectations,
Standards and validations
That reciprocate and duplicate
Patterns of self-hatred

I no longer want to be dictated
Forced under a cookie cutter, alternated, tweaked, and adjusted
My body, my mind wants to be liberated!

– Note to self

21.

Self-Acceptance: An Unfinished, Intergenerational Story

Judy Verseghy

If I'm to be honest, I don't remember all that much about being young. Most of the time has just passed by me, leaving vague recollections and fleeting feelings. Most of my vivid memories revolve around my fear and disgust of my own body and my desire to contain this mass that seemed uncontrollable, stretching far beyond the space that it was allowed to occupy.

I remember being four and wearing a size 6x shirt, realizing that 6x was the size for a six-year-old, and already feeling like I had somehow done something wrong, as though an extra inch of fabric made me an outsider—marked me as an uncontrollable body. I remember being nine and stepping on a scale that read 120 pounds and vowing to myself not to gain any more, no matter how much taller I got or how much my body wanted to fill out in different ways.

For years, I was plagued by my thighs. I would look down at them when I sat in a seat, or on the floor, and gaze in disgust as they pooled their way outwards. Once, I was sitting on the floor of my high school with my legs crossed, and a dear friend of mine grabbed the inside of my knee (which had been exposed by a very 90's large hole in my jeans), spread my calf and thigh apart, pointed out the way the flesh met in the middle, surrounded by a volume of skin and fat, and said, "Look, it's like a butt crack!" She thought it was hilarious. I was mortified. Another friend, another time, asked me why my thighs looked like cottage cheese while we were in the middle of class.

These were the off-the-cuff, lighthearted messages I was getting from the people I loved and who loved me. These statements were the nice version of the jeers from people on the street or the clothing store salespeople asking if I wanted things in a larger size as they looked me up and down. And, honestly, these little comments hurt more and made me feel more like an aberrant outsider than the comments from strangers ever did. It's weird, actually, how the people who loved me most and made the kindest, most seemingly innocuous comments were the ones who cut the deepest.

"You have such a pretty face!" my mother would tell me frequently. I remember that these words came out most often in the context of my being upset that my sister had gotten the looks in the family. Petite, slim, and with gorgeous and natural strawberry blonde hair and bright blue eyes, she was always the one that was complimented for being so very beautiful by visiting family and friends. I was primarily known for being kind and smart, which I suppose was a good thing, and I am grateful that my mother always told me how much she loved my brains and my heart (and my pretty face). But I always wanted to be beautiful because I knew that that's where a girl's real value lay.

In telling me how pretty my face was, my mother was clearly trying to make me feel better. What I heard in that message though was her telling me that my body, by comparison, wasn't pretty. She would encourage me to watch what I ate or to swim, which she always told me made my legs looks nice. When I would confront her about how these comments made me feel—how I felt the weight of her disapproval and how I needed her to stop making me feel like I was simultaneously less than and too much—she would cry, and I would back down. She was only concerned for my health, she said. And I believed her. And I still do believe her—that her concern is that I am unhealthy and that I will die early or become chronically ill with arthritis, which runs in the family, or diabetes, the scourge of fat folks everywhere. I just don't agree that her premonitions will come true.

My mother's words came from a place of love. They stemmed from years of being taught about the importance of maintaining a healthy weight—something that she could not do as a child, as she was so slim that she was placed in special programs at school that had the goal of fattening children up. She told me that the school staff who were monitoring her would give her full fat milk and a generous portion of carbohydrates and be dismayed when her body would not reap the dividends in the form of added padding. Her body was policed, like mine—two kids on very different ends of a very short spectrum of acceptable weights and sizes. I feel badly for her child self, as I do for mine, having to live in the knowledge that our bodies were unacceptable, each for being what the other was not.

Now, at age thirty-three and size twenty-four, I have made peace with my body. I found the fat activist movement, read about health at every size, and finally stopped deconstructing every little or large lump and bump in the mirror every day. Some days, sure, I feel down about being a fat woman. But, mostly, I revel in it, reclaiming the title fat as a personal and political identity and defying anyone who dares to deride this tremendous vessel I call my body. It took a long time to move from one point to another along the spectrum of self-love, and although I can't say I've fully arrived, I'm certainly feeling much better than when I was young and put myself on one diet after another, only to hate my unwieldy body even more when the diets didn't work. Yet now I face a new challenge, in the form of relaying my hard-won self-acceptance to my young children.

I thought that by being a fat woman who had applied a critical lens to uncover the social construction of fatness, I could protect my children from feeling the same self-hatred that I did as a child. So, when my kids were born, I vetoed Barbies, did my best to avoid commercials, and gave messages about how wonderful all of our bodies are, including their differences. I thought with a concerted effort I could shield my beautiful kids from the damning messages that tell them that thin is the only beautiful and that being beautiful is the only worth. But I can't.

I remember when my middle child was just five years old, lying on the bed with me while I folded laundry, saying "I wish my belly were smaller." My stomach dropped to the ground, knowing, just knowing, that this was the beginning of years' worth of discussions.

So, we talk. We talk for years because parenting is an endless opportunity for discussion. We talk of self-love and fat hate. We talk body positivity and media literacy. We stay up late into the night discussing privilege and patriarchy and body politics.

We talk about appreciating our bodies and appearances, listing the things we love about ourselves. And we talk about all the things that we don't love so much and how body positivity and self-acceptance are not a steady accumulation achieved by repeating mantras. Some days, no matter how hard you try, you still can't get over your belly that juts out over your pants or your thighs that jiggle when you walk.

Some days, my child tells me, they hate their body. Most days, they say.

I talk about how I felt the same way. More than twenty years wasted, feeling bad about myself not as a consequence of my own flaws but of other people's lack of acceptance.

I work even harder to save my children from this misery.

I become friends with an amazing group of rad fat women. We talk feminism and fat activism and self-love and body positivity. I am refreshed. I affectionately dub them my fat girls, and my little ones are taken with them even before they meet.

One sunny summer day, we begin what becomes a 'big fat beach day' annual tradition. We claim our space. We are unapologetic as we bask in the sun, flesh unbound and glistening. We eat baguettes and grapes and tarts, and we sneer at the bros who laugh and point as they walk by because fuck them and their beauty ideals. When we get too hot, we make our way to the water, cooling ourselves as we move our bodies around, as though we are bouncing along the surface of the moon.

It is glorious.

My kids and I return home and talk often about these wonderful women and this amazing day, and how lucky we are to have a team of strong models of self-love. I am confident that we have turned a corner and that these years of discussions have finally made their way somewhere; they have successfully fought off the endless cacophony of voices that screams at my children that they must have 'perfect' bodies in order to be worthy of love and respect. Well done, mama. You have fought the good fight and won. Or so I thought. But the challenges of parenting are not so easily met. The clamour of hateful voices cannot, it turns out, be extinguished by a single, perfect day at the beach.

Three months later, while watching their favourite star on YouTube, my baby casually says, without making eye contact, "I've stopped eating my entire lunch and put myself on a diet. I've lost ten pounds!"

My heart drops.

22.

Braced

Sam Abel

REACTIONS

I am someone who used to frequently get a lot of crap in public for my body.

ha, what an ugly cow.
stupid whale.
hahahaha look at that fat bitch!
hahaha
She's just sitting there! Let's throw something!
POP

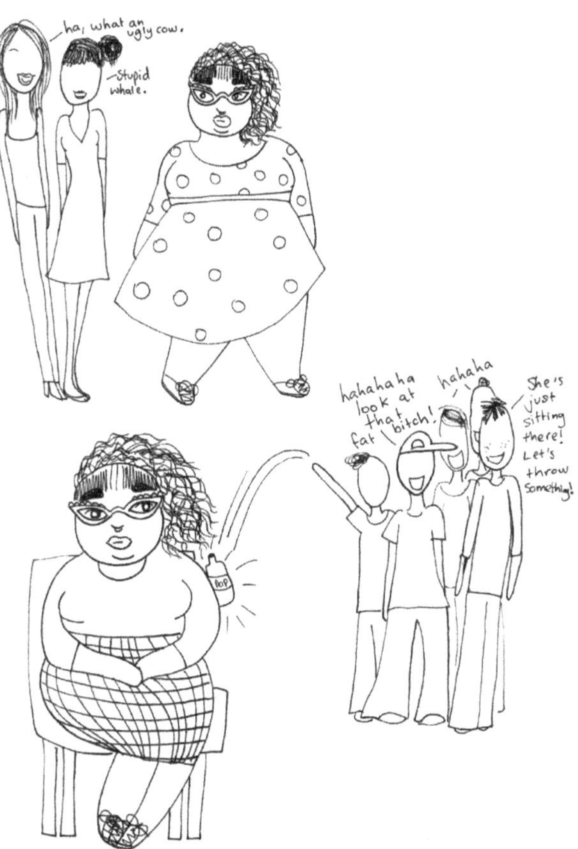

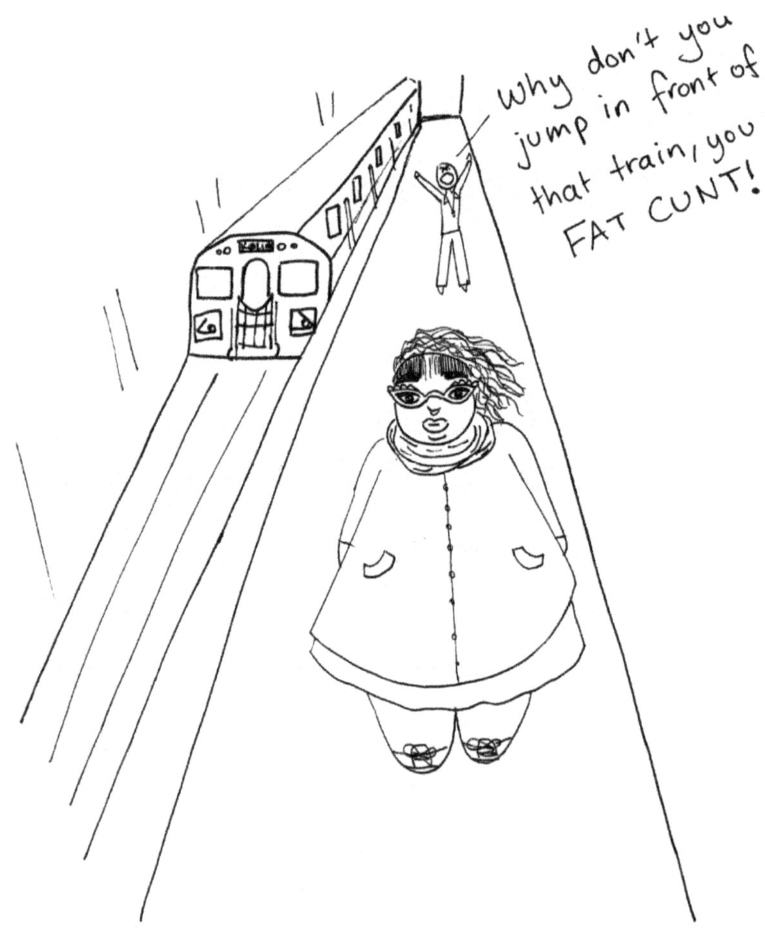
Why don't you
jump in front of
that train, you
FAT CUNT!

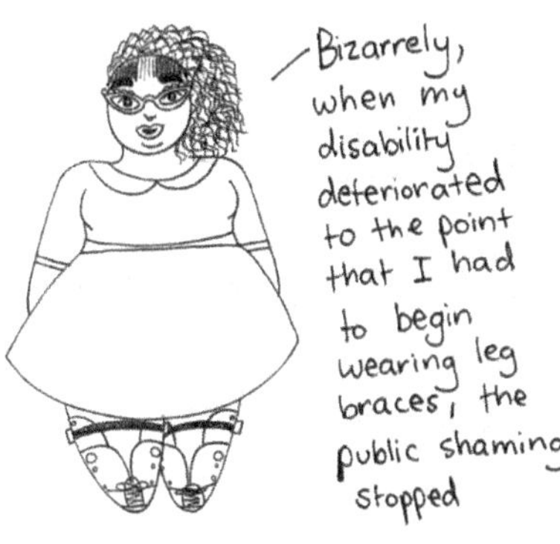
Bizarrely, when my disability deteriorated to the point that I had to begin wearing leg braces, the public shaming stopped

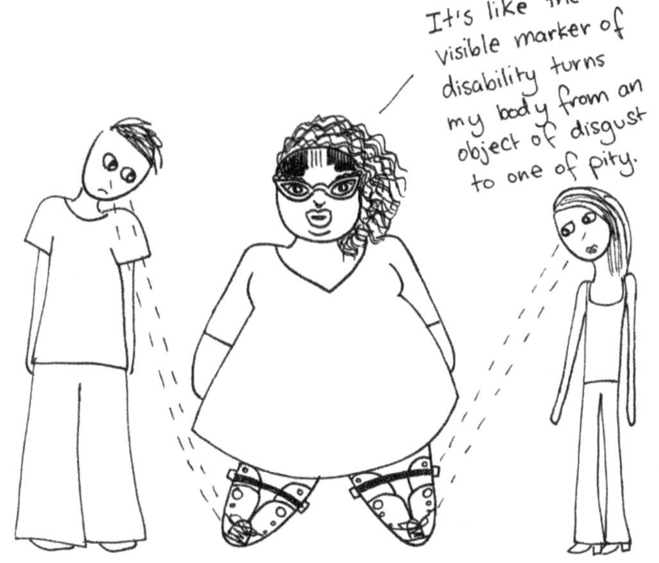
It's like the visible marker of disability turns my body from an object of disgust to one of pity.

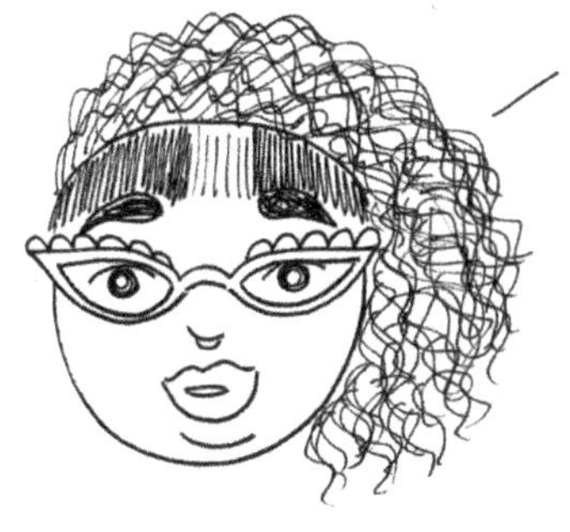
It's totally disorienting and I'm not sure what to feel about it.

HAUNTED

I have always been fat.

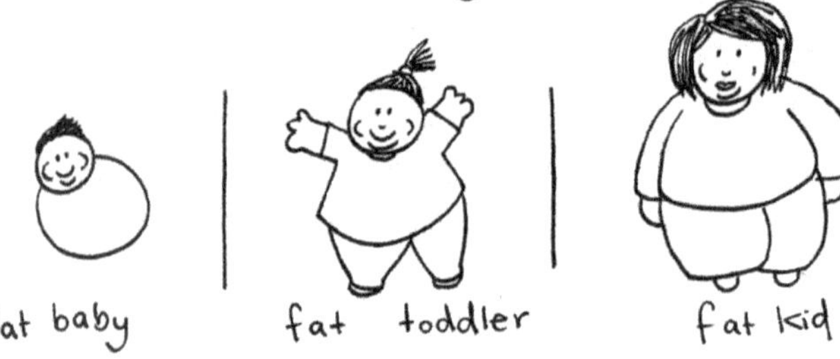

Like most fat people (especially women-identified ones), I have had a long and difficult journey with my body. When I first found the fat acceptance movement I began to see that my struggles were not singular or my fault. This helped me to mostly move past hate & blame, and into acceptance and peace.

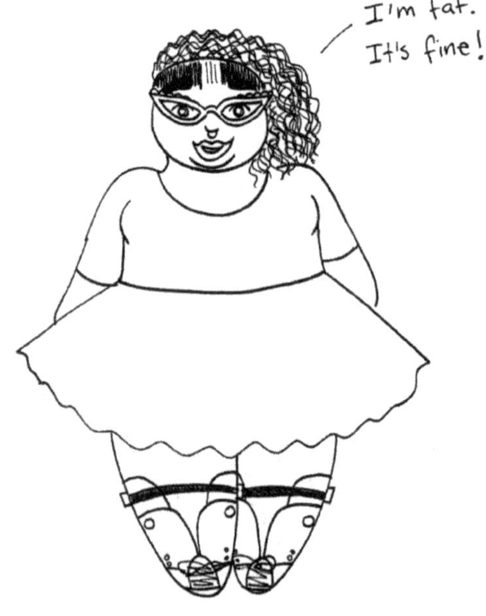

However, since my disability began impacting me in more profound and debilitating ways (the last 6 years or so), I have gained about 60lbs.

Me in 2009
Me in 2016
So I now have super complicated feelings about my fatness that are intertwined with my anger at my increasing pain & dwindling mobility

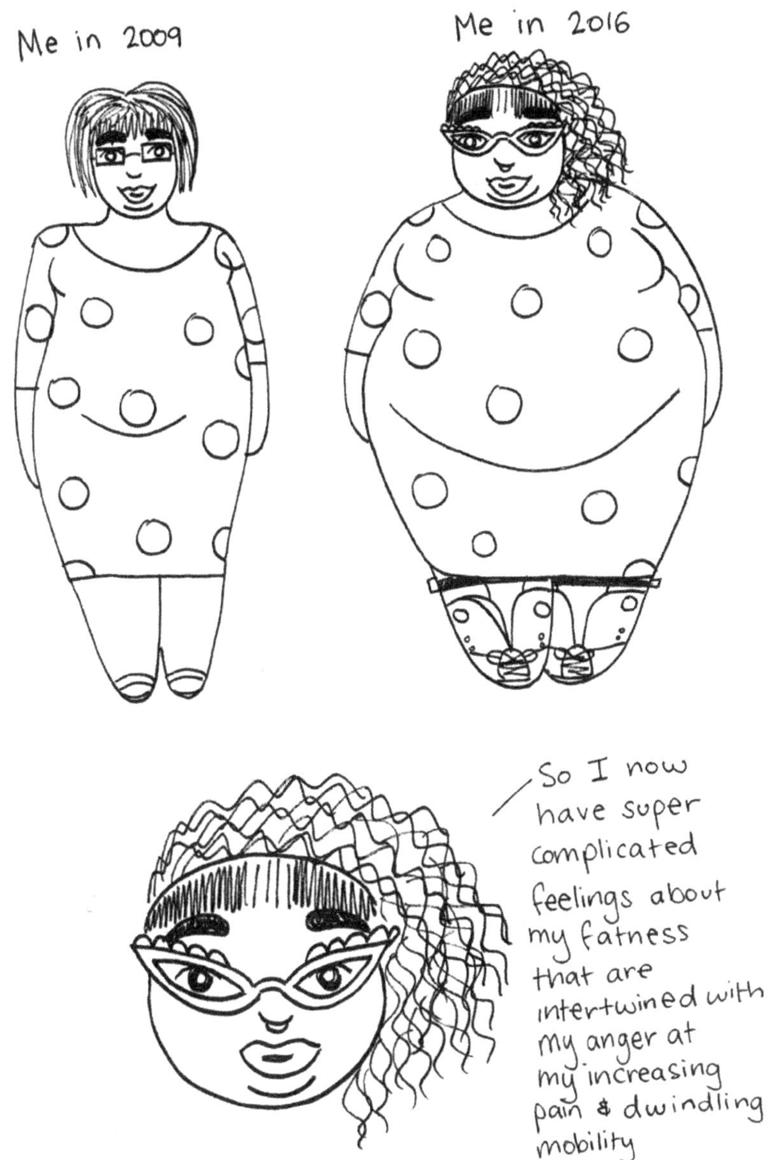

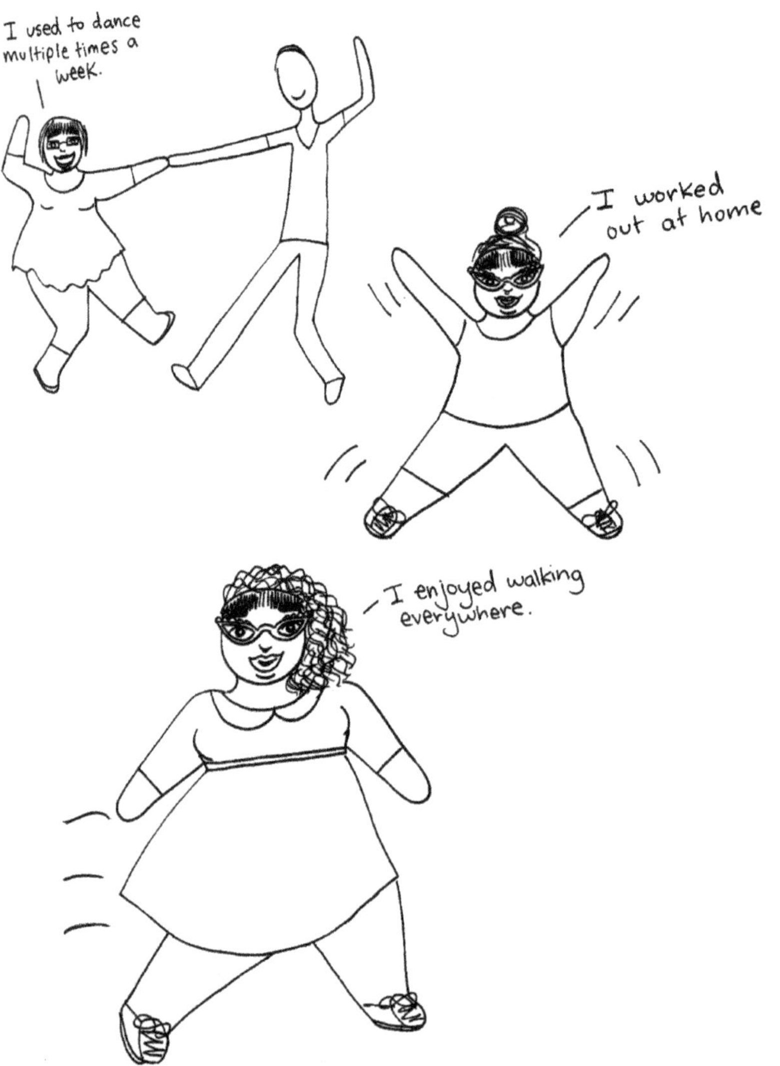
Because while I was always fat,
I was also always active.
I used to dance multiple times a week.
I worked out at home
I enjoyed walking everywhere.

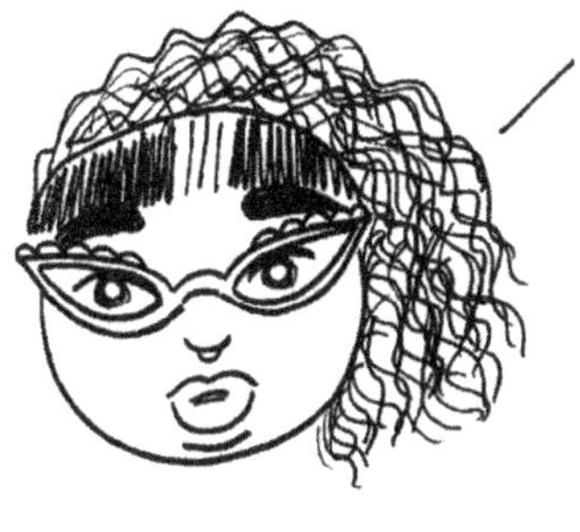

The last time I danced...

I spent 45 minutes struggling (as opposed to when I could easily dance for 4-5 hours)

It took me FIVE DAYS to recover.

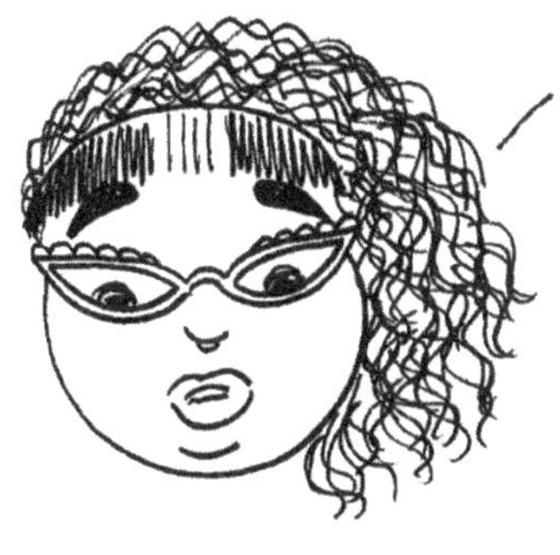

I stopped dancing, fading away from something that had once been so important.

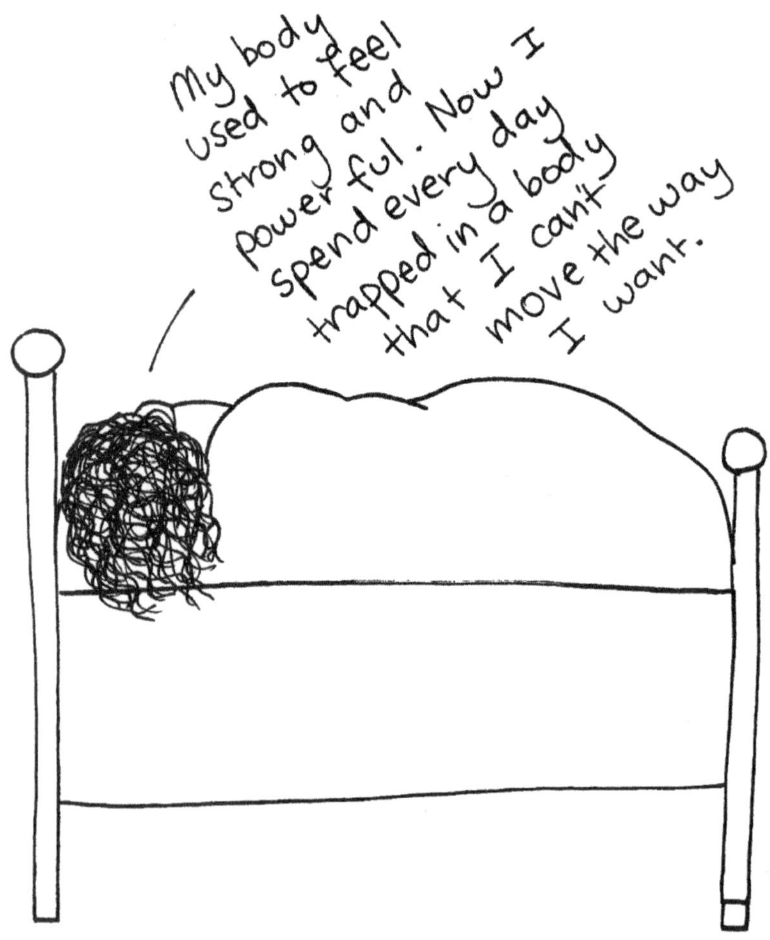
My body used to feel strong and powerful. Now I spend every day trapped in a body that I can't move the way I want.

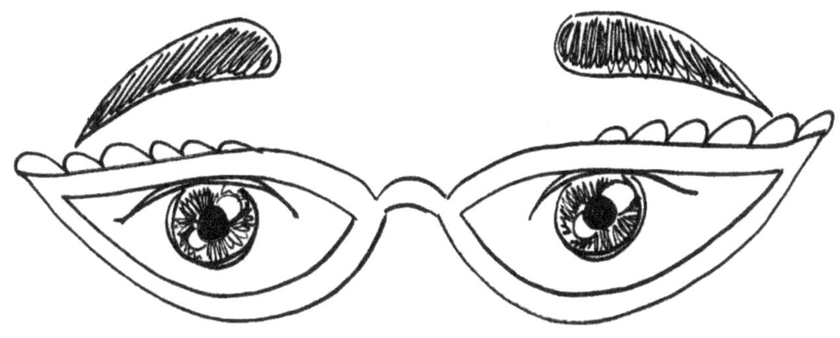

I AM HAUNTED
BY THE PERSON
I USED TO BE.

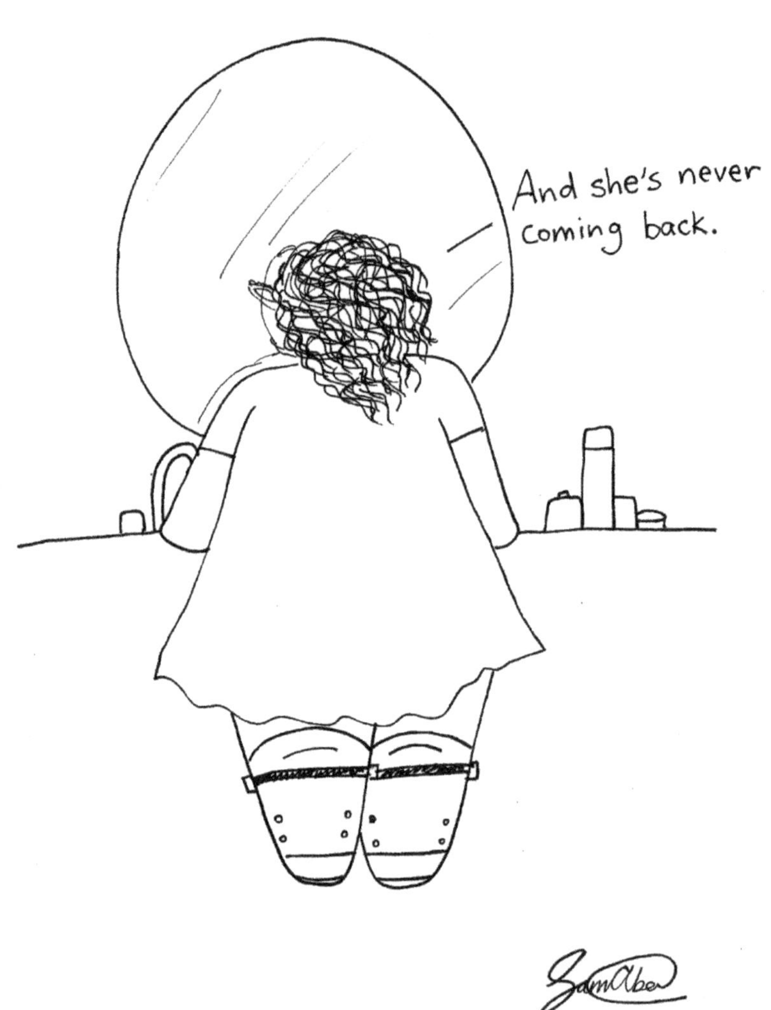
And she's never
coming back.

23.

Lessons Learned from Fat Women on Television

Idil Abdillahi and May Friedman

What happens when we choose to take our theoretical focus and turn towards a sphere that is meant to be beneath analysis?

We are fat, racialized academics. In our scholarly work, we've learned how to talk about healthism, about discourses of normativity, and about the aesthetic oppression of fat phobia. But these analyses don't stop when we lie down on the sofa and switch on a television show, which, it must be owned, we love to do. In this chapter, we aim to unpack and connect our leisure time pursuits with our academic knowledge by considering the ways that we have learned about fat bodies that we see on television.

Although this discussion takes up specific examples of fat in popular culture, the lessons we've learned have been offered to us through hours of engagement with different media—YouTube clips, subway advertisements, tweets and posts, and other artefacts. The messages we hear about fat bodies, both our own and those of others, are varied and intersected, but the core truths we explore here have resonated for us across multiple platforms. We offer these specific instances, then, as merely a few key examples of lessons that we are learning and relearning every day. Importantly, we don't offer these lessons as evidence that engagement with popular culture is wrong (Friedman; Boylorn; Kavka). We see our immersion in popular culture as both inevitable and necessary (Pozner), and, truthfully, we're not breaking up with Netflix anytime soon. Instead, we aim to be critical consumers of culture considering the ways that popular culture contributes to how we understand the world and ourselves.

Lesson One: Good Fatties Only, Please

Our initial reaction in seeing Whitney Way Thore's video of her as "A Fat Woman Dancing" was relief to see a super-sized woman doing something that is generally viewed as forbidden—or impossible—for very fat bodies. We were equally heartened to see Whitney's internet celebrity translated into her TLC television show, *My Big Fat, Fabulous Life*. Although we continue to feel that Thore makes a positive contribution to popular culture as a generally happy and optimistic woman of size, her story also reveals the extent of the stigma experienced by fat women in showing the hatred and shaming she experiences as she moves in the world. Yet for all that we're encouraged by the inclusion of a story like Whitney's as a necessary antidote to such horrible offerings as *My 600LB Life*—and for all that, we'd love to have her over to dinner (stop by if you're around, Whitney! We'll bake you a cake!)—we are also suspicious of the conditions that permit this particular woman to transgress the limitations imposed on fat women in the public sphere.

Whitney exemplifies the trope of the "good fatty" (Bias). With few exceptions, she is extremely careful about her food intake, and she is consistently shown as motivated to partake in exercise and dance. In other words, Whitney interrupts expectations of fat people as inactive overeaters. On the one hand, this interruption is welcome in diffusing tired stereotypes; on the other, thinking of Whitney this way suggests that people who are fat because they like to eat fat foods or because they are uninterested in exercise deserve the stigma of fatphobia. In defending her own experiences, Whitney's story, perhaps through no fault of her own, places other fatties at risk of comparison.

The notion of Whitney as a good fatty is taken even further through the implication that her fat body is due to polycystic ovarian syndrome (PCOS), a metabolic condition. Whitney's frequent explanations about PCOS certainly remind viewers that fat arrives for many reasons and may be difficult to shift, but we worry this may come at the cost of throwing "bad" fatties under the bus. In addition, the discussion of PCOS moves Whitney from being someone who deserves to be hated to someone who becomes a mascot, a valiant object of pity who struggles through adversity. We're reminded that being a fatty, whether good or bad, ultimately sucks.

Whitney's ability to perform as a good fatty requires access to privilege, which may also explain why she is able to stand (and dance!) as the poster child for fat living. Whitney can spend countless hours on body management because she is supported financially by her wealthy parents. She is college educated and has had the cultural capital to explore employment in a range of settings, including internationally (Thore). Finally, Whitney's white skin and uncontested access to class privilege, as well as her overall health and ability, position her as a very specific fat woman who can escape from the intersections that racism, ableism, and classism may inject into fat phobia.

Lesson Two: No Love Lost

Fat bodies are given a different treatment in another TLC offering, *90-Day Fiancé*.[1] The premise of the show involves an American citizen who partners with someone from outside the United States. Permitted entry on a special premarriage visa, the immigrating partner must get married within ninety days or leave the country. The specific matching of culturally diverse couples on this show leads to a range of issues ripe for exploration, but we will confine our analysis in this section to considering the show's treatment of fat people.

Although this show represents a departure from much popular culture by presenting fat people as marriageable or romantically relevant at all, it maintains some core assumptions about love and fatness. Specifically, the show takes for granted that fat people are unlovable, both because of their grotesque aesthetic, but also by alluding to stereotypes such as the laziness, gluttony, and lack of self control of fat people. As viewers, we are dismayed, though not surprised, to see that the couples that include larger people are generally devoid of any romance or sexuality and are instead presented as hostile, pitiable business arrangements; unsurprisingly, these relationships generally fall apart fairly quickly. While other partnerships are fuelled by love, sex, and drama, these specific pairings are presented in more unromantic ways. Unable to perform as lovable people, the fat American members of these couples must provide stability, financial support, and access to an

American life (presumed to be a benefit) to offset their unappealing bodies. This is most obvious in the case of George, a fat man who is engaged to a (thin) foreign bride.

It is important to note that fat protagonists on *90-Day Fiancé* are white. Specifically, the construction of a pitiable white subject, even one who is reviled, is predicated on whiteness. Notably, the fiancés of the two fat American women on season four were racialized men from so-called developing nations. The show seems to suggest, without much subtlety, that fat Americans, as damaged goods, need to look for partnership among people who are equally marginal, offering the status of Americanness as a carrot to tempt attractive but impoverished foreigners. The racism and colonial dynamic of these interactions are deeply troubling.

Even as fat Americans are presented as simultaneously subhuman (but better than non-Americans nonetheless), tropes of poverty in both foreign and American contexts emerge. In one case, Tunisian fiancé Mohamed was presented as cruel to Danielle, his American fiancée, because of his frustration at finding that her (working-class) life was not as he had expected. The relationship between Danielle and Mohamed rests at the intersection of racism, classism, and fatphobia, with the Orientalizing of Mohamed casting him as a cartoon villain at the same time that Danielle's overcrowded mobile home is fetishized. The show presents a gaze that simultaneously reviles Danielle for being fat and poor and condemns Mohamed (who is himself cast as the impoverished "Third World" subject) for making the same judgment. The relationship eventually degrades into a courtroom drama with neither party being presented sympathetically. Although this example (and many like it in this show) does not examine the specific intersection of race and fatness on the same body, racism is implicated in the treatment of fatness. By framing both fat and foreignness as undesirable and unattractive, the show maintains and extends stereotypes of poverty, fat, whiteness, and racialization.

Lesson Three: Fat, Black, and Absent

Given the examples that we've given above, it is perhaps unsurprising, though nonetheless disheartening, that we found ourselves struggling for examples of fat Black female characters on television. Although fat women's bodies were hardly overrepresented in the popular culture we consume, we found examples across virtually all genres and eras. When we sought out fat female bodies that were Black or racialized, however, our conversation dried up. We acknowledge that there are a few such roles—Mercedes on the hit show *Glee*, notable for being one of few characters on the show to never establish a long-term romantic relationship; the brief but tremendously interesting visibility of Veronica "Pooh" Poleate on *She's In Charge*; and the gross overrepresentation of fat Black folk on weight loss shows—but overall, we were disappointed, though unsurprised, by the lack of women who look, quite frankly, like us. Where were our fat Brown and Black representatives? And what could we make of their absence?

Perhaps casting directors avoid inclusion of fat Black women out of fear of perpetuating the Mammy stereotype (Hill Collins)? Although we'd like to give the television industry that much credit, the enduring popularity of other stereotypical Black femininities—the angry Black woman and the hypersexualized Jezebel—does not support this view. Instead, we'd like to suggest that the relative absence of Black fat female bodies in popular television shows the limits of bodily transgression; in short, to be simultaneously fat, Black, and female is to be, literally and figuratively, too much. Going even further, Sonia Renee Taylor argues that fat Black bodies are equally excised from discussions of body positivity, suggesting for all their invisibility in the public sphere, fat Black women are expected and, therefore, not radical. As Taylor states: "Being seen in our bodies, in our fullness and beauty is a birthright women of color have never had ... even beginning to dismantle weight stigma is to be seen as fully human in this society. Far too often, that is a privilege that requires white skin and no matter how much I weigh or how naked I get, I will never have that." The outcome—that fat Black women are too much to be included but too normative to be celebrated as revolutionary—is deeply saddening.

Conclusion

We began by defending our engagement with popular culture, and despite our many reservations and frustrations with the ways that bodies like ours are presented (and not presented) in popular media, we can't see ourselves changing our habits anytime soon. Yet it would be false to present our engagement with popular culture as solely passive. We consider Jennifer Pozner's challenge that "Structural changes are needed to achieve the creative, diverse, challenging media we all deserve, and we're going to have to fight for such shifts" (325-26). Our relationship with media is constantly shifting. We use our classrooms to unpack and critically engage with various media. We use the multi-modal and endlessly dialogic platforms of internet spaces to support, shift, exhaust, infuriate, and otherwise extend our understanding of what we see and read. Finally, we are ourselves engaged in media making in both small and large ways (*It Takes a Riot*).

As cultural critics, we do not understand culture to be some highbrow offering beyond us; we also reject the notion of culture as our unique selling point—our Blackness/Brownness, our ethnicness somehow rendering us cultured folks. Instead, we see culture as the world around us, the endless sea of messages that we swim through, the stereotypes and ugly talk, but also the beautiful and revolutionary corners. We would like to see a world with more room for fatness and specifically a more nuanced, complex, and layered view of fat bodies of all races, genders, classes, sexualities, and abilities, but we're mindful that this shift comes from us. Our talking and teaching and writing and engagement with the world at large change the story of fat and that, in turn, changes our stories about ourselves in a recursive and endless loop. Our guilty pleasures produce some of our most cogent critiques and our awareness of what is included and what is left out help equip us to become part of a transgressive revolution. We hope you'll join us!

Endnotes

1. Although we have consumed many hours of *90-Day Fiancé*, our analysis here centres on season four.

Works Cited

90-Day Fiancé. Directed by Jessica Hernandez and Kevin Rhoades, 2014, TLC.

Boylorn, Robin M. "As Seen on TV: An Autoethnographic Reflection on Race and Reality Television." *Critical Studies in Media Communication,* vol. 25 no. 4, 2008, pp. 413-33.

Bias, Stacy. "12 Good Fatty Archetypes." *StacyBias.net,* June 2014.

Friedman, May. "Survivor Skills: Authenticity, Representation, and Why I Want to Teach Reality TV." *Dialogue: The Interdisciplinary Journal of Popular Culture and Pedagogy,* vol. 2, no. 1, 2014, journaldialogue.org/issues/issue-2/survivor-skills-authenticity-representation-and-why-i-want-to-teach-reality-tv/. Accessed 7 Oct. 2020.

Hill Collins, Patricia. *Black Feminist Thought: Knowledge, Consciousness and the Politics of Empowerment.* 2nd ed. Routledge, 2000.

It Takes a Riot: Race, Rebellion and Reform. Directed by Howard Grandison, executive producers Idil Abdillahi, Simon Black, and Howard Grandison, 2017.

Kavka, Misha. *Reality TV.* Edinburgh University Press, 2012.

Pozner, Jennifer L. *Reality Bites Back: The Troubling Truth about Guilty Pleasure TV.* Seal Press, 2004.

My Big Fat Fabulous Life. Directed by Keith Koslov, 2015, TLC.

Taylor, Sonia Renee. "Weighting to Be Seen: Being Fat, Black, and Invisible in Body Positivity." *The Body is Not an Apology,* 9 Apr. 2017, thebodyisnotanapology.com/magazine/weighting-to-be-seen-being-fat-black-and-invisible-in-body-positivity/. Accessed 7 Oct. 2020.

Thore, Whitney Way. "I Do It with the Lights On: And 10 More Discoveries on the Road to a Blissfully Shame-Free Life." Ballantine Books, 2016.

24.

Embodied: The Female Body as a Repository of Experience

Leesa Streifler

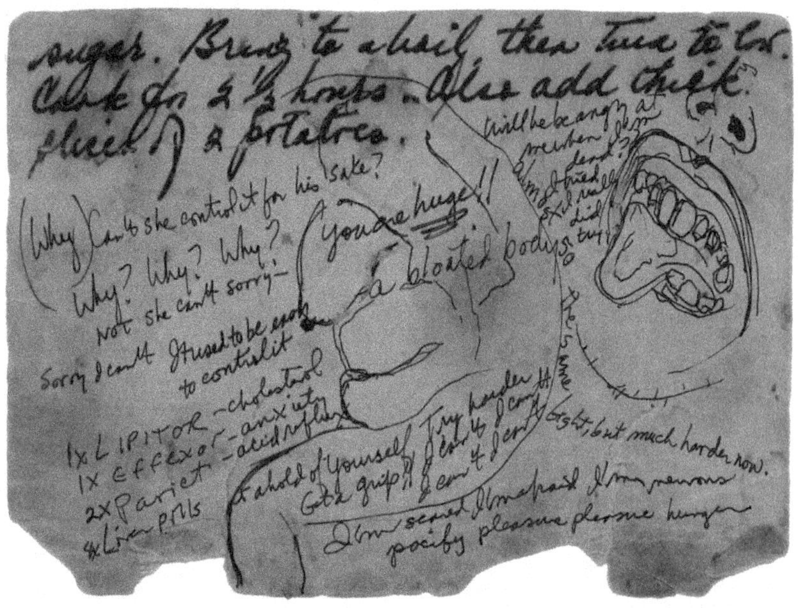

"Her Domain: A Recipe Card Series" 2006, 25" x 38"; 63.50 cm x 96.52 cm; Chromogenic print based on drawing on existing recipe card.

This work is part of a series of twelve works based on my mother-in-law's recipe cards, which I inherited after she passed away in 2005. I was attracted initially to the beauty of her penmanship and the beautiful golden colour and irregular edges of the cards. Conceptually,

I began thinking about what the ubiquitous recipe card represents. It is a document that holds much more importance than just instructions for cooking a certain mealtime dish. My intention for this work is to highlight the importance of recipe cards as significant documents. Normally dismissed as part of the invisible and unappreciated labour of women in the home, I wanted to raise awareness of the foundational place of recipe cards as signifiers of the sustenance of family provided by women. I became a mother in 2003, and my writing reflects my corporeal identity at the time, including the medications I was on and my battle with stress-eating and negative body image. The dialogue is based on my feelings of guilt in relation to being a mother struggling with body issues. The male I refer to in this image is my son who was five years old at the time.

The work opposite utilizes me as the subject and is intended to critique the dominant male perspective regarding fat women. The woman in this work is asserting her self-acceptance and instructing the male viewer to take responsibility for his misguided feelings regarding the female body.

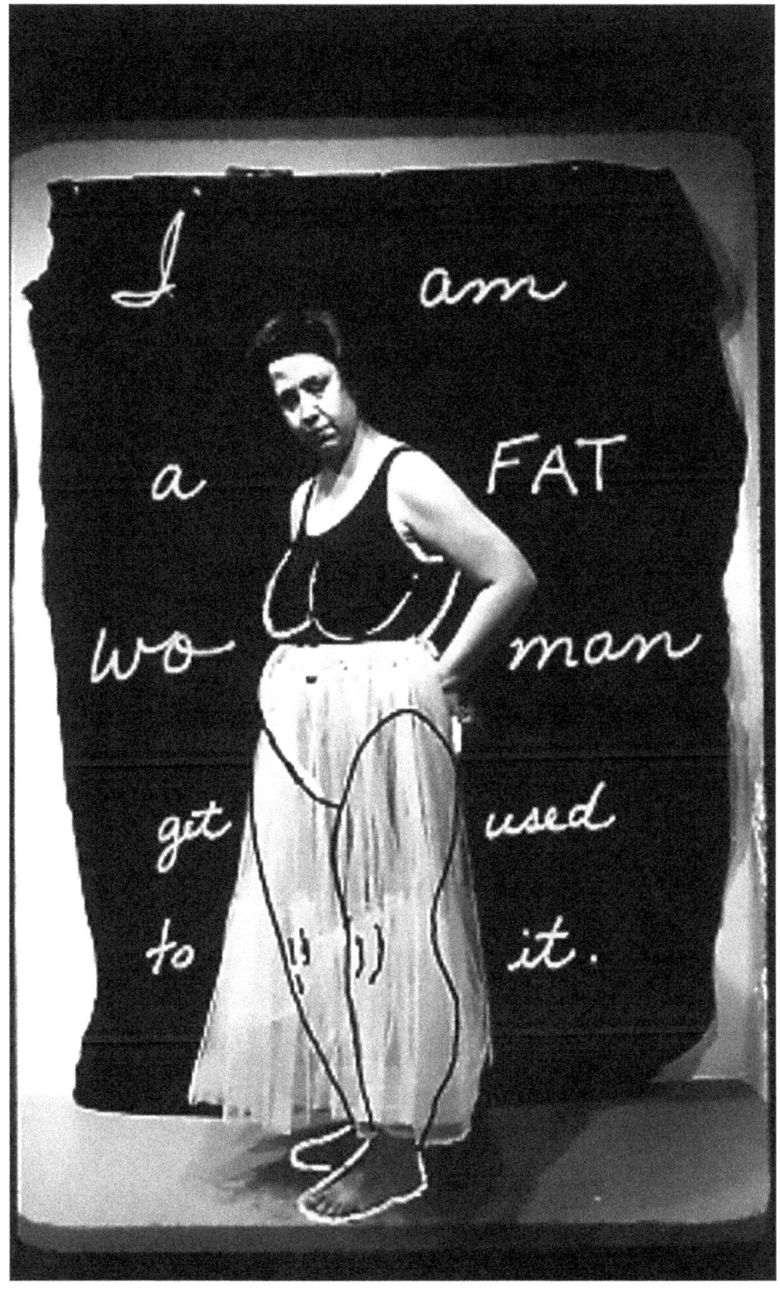

"Adaptation" from NORMAL series, 1992-1997, 7" x 5"; 17.78 x 12.7 cm, white marker on silverprint.

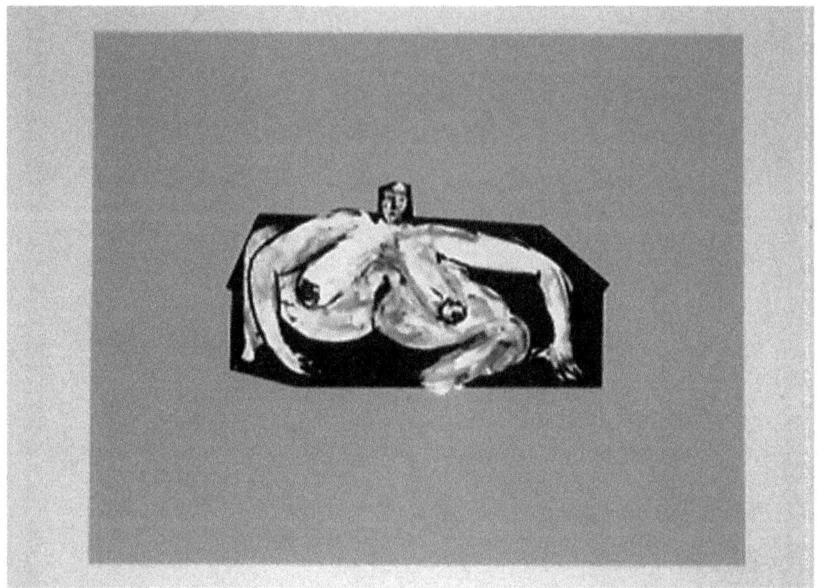

"Contained" 2003, 25 x 38"; 63.50 x 96.52 cm; Chromogenic print

This work is part of a series exploring suburban domesticity. I had just moved into a split-level home in the suburbs and was feeling overwhelmed by the expectations that I imagined were upon me. I feared being stifled by these expectations and that I would not fit this lifestyle.

25.

Like It or Not: A Dose of Fat Activism for the Medical Community

Cat Pausé

My friend, Gabrielle, has a tenuous relationship with the medical profession. Like many women, she has been subjected to condescending discussions around her diet, exercise, and weight from health professionals who don't bother to take the time to learn anything about her health behaviors but simply reprimand her for not doing enough to ensure her body mass index (BMI) falls into the normal category. She had established a relationship with a particular doctor, who tolerated her refusal to be weighed but still subjected her to unsolicited nonsense about her body. One day, she found herself in the unfortunate situation of needing a refill on her inhaler prescription while in the middle of an asthma attack. She sought care at her doctor's office, only to have her request be denied unless she agreed to be weighed. Here she was, standing in the middle of the office, struggling to breathe, and being told that unless she got onto the scale, the refill would not be provided.

Gabrielle's story is not uncommon—fat people who seek medical care are often subjected to the antifat attitudes of their providers (Foster et al. 168; Pausé, "Die" 135). Due to the antifat attitudes of their healthcare providers, fat people have limited access to evidenced based healthcare that is practiced in an environment free of stigma (Lee and Pausé, "Stigma in Practice").

They are regularly stigmatized by their healthcare providers (Puhl and Heuer 1022; Teachman and Brownell 1530), resulting in poorer care and even reduced access to healthcare (Budd et al. 131; Carryer 94; Drury et al. 557; Puhl and Heuer 958); fat patients often receive substandard care (Amy et al. 152). Healthcare providers may rely more on body size to judge physical health than other diagnostic tools or even their client's own information and perceptions (Persky and Eccleston 730).

What are the ways that we, as fat studies scholars and as fat activists, can combat these antifat attitudes and fight for quality, evidenced-based medical care? One way we can do this is to educate healthcare providers (Hague and White 58; Maroney and Golub 388). Like the general public, much of the antifat bias held by those in the medical profession stems from ignorance about fatness. Many people believe that their family doctor is a knowledgeable person around issues of weight and health. I would refute that. Most general practitioners have had very little education in nutrition (Adams et al. 3). Very few have an appreciation for the social construction of health and medicine. It is very unlikely that they have had any kind of training to providing effective care to fat patients (Bocquier et al. 787; Kristeller and Hoerr 544). And it is even more unlikely that they regularly read the scientific journals that publish cutting-edge research and understanding around issues of weight and health; most spend two hours or less a week reading current research and evidence of best practice (Mukohara and Schwartz 405). If they were practicing evidenced-based healthcare, they would never prescribe weight loss as a treatment for any patient.

I began educating health and social providers on the obesity myths in my second year in New Zealand. The title of my workshop has varied; I've called it "Unpacking the Obesity Myths" and "Big Fat Facts." For a few months, in tribute to charlatans like Dr. Oz, I gave it a subtitle, "Big Fat Facts: What You Don't Know about What Isn't Killing You." The workshops are prepared and delivered at the invitation of groups, including hospitals, museums, university campuses, and local rotary clubs.

I begin by introducing myself as a fat person as well as both a fat studies scholar and a fat activist. I share some highlights of my work and the underlying goals that drive me. Fat people deserve the same rights and dignity as nonfat people; fat people also deserve to receive evidenced-based healthcare free from shame and provider bias. I suggest that we live in a fatphobic world, and I share some examples of fat hatred and fat shaming in action. I discuss how we find antifat attitudes in children as young as three (Cramer and Steinwert, 440) and how young people would rather date a felon than a fat person (Crandall and Biernat, 237). I encourage them to pay attention to the examples of fat hatred and shaming in their own lives. I ask them to provide reasons why we are so afraid of fat—and the list is generally what you would expect. Most people talk about health and diabetes; wanting to be active and able to do the things they want to do. Very rarely do they talk about the aesthetics involved or that being fat is gross and disgusting. But you can feel it in the room—under the surface—the things they aren't ready to say out loud (especially to a fat person).

We then move into the second part of the workshop, and we consider the reasons that we are afraid of fat. I propose three main reasons: morality, intersectionality, and ignorance.

Simply put, slim bodies are good bodies, and fat bodies are bad bodies (and reflect the morality of the person who embodies said good or bad body). Drawing on the work of Annemarie Jutel ("Weighing Health"; "Does Size Really Matter"), I suggest that we believe we are able to read bodies. A slim body is an active body and a successful body—a body that suggests willpower and discipline, all qualities of a good person within a Judeo-Christian moral framework. A fat body, in contrast, is an inactive body and a lazy body—a body that suggests a lack of willpower and discipline, all qualities of a bad person, within this same framework. Therefore, slim people are good people, and fat people are bad people (Pausé, "Rebel Heart").

Another reason I propose is the intersection of body size with issues of gender, race, and class. Paul Campos suggests that antifat attitudes are often poorly masked attitudes about race and class—a way for individuals to indulge in their racism, classism, and sexism without acknowledging those feelings (85). Although I strongly dispute any notion that antifat attitudes are the last socially acceptable form of prejudice, I do believe that exploring how body size and our attitudes around body size are shaped by our attitudes around race, class, and gender is an important part of understanding antifat attitudes and the lived experiences of fat people (and how they are not a homogenous population). A great way to illustrate this with a group is to engage in an exercise created by the flabulous fat activist, Marilyn Wann ("Weight of the Nation"). Using a whiteboard, you begin by asking the audience to suggest characteristics and stereotypes of fat and slim people. (Make sure to reassure them that you understand that they do not believe these things to be true; they are more advanced than that, but these are commonly held beliefs of others, of those people out there). Once you have that list, replace the words "slim" and "fat" with "rich" and "poor" and ask if the list still fits. More than likely, it does. Next, and this is where it will get uncomfortable, replace the words "slim/rich" and "fat/poor" with "white" and "Black." I use the words Pakeha and Māori when working with a New Zealand audience. (This is usually a good place to remind them that this is not about what they believe.)

~~Slim Rich~~ Pakeha	**~~Fat Poor~~ Māori**
Smart	Unhealthy
Happy	Inactive
Active	Lazy
Healthy	Dumb
Attractive	Unsuccessful
Successful	Sad
Motivated	Ugly/Gross

I ask again if the list still fits. And I'm usually met with silence. Deafening, uncomfortable silence. If there is a nonwhite person in the room, they are often quick to speak up and confirm that the list still fits. With that allowance, the silent individuals will usually join in agreement or at least provide some head nods. On select occasions, someone (usually a middle-aged white person) will scoff at this and dismiss it as the "way it used to be." They will suggest we have moved forward (ah yes, our postracial world!), and that this does not represent how people think today. This is usually a lone voice in the crowd, and I've always wondered if this person has now dismissed my entire message based on this dissonance; perhaps, they were never on board with me to begin with. Before I move on from this section, I speak again about the intersections of oppression and caution them against conflating, or equating, these categories (ethnicity, class, and body size). Understanding intersectionality is much more than reducing individuals into single groups and much more than simply adding groups on (Pausé "Process" 82). The last reason for fatphobia is ignorance. I like to ask my audience to work in small groups to determine whether they believe the following statements are true or false:

- The BMI is a good measure of morbidity and mortality.
- Being fat is unhealthy.
- There are safe and permanent ways for people to lose weight.

After allowing them time to chat about them with their neighbors, I propose to them that they are all false and constitute what I call "the obesity myths." We then go through the evidence that refutes these common myths, and I point out information that has contributed to the myths. For example, we consider the often cited three hundred thousand deaths a year in the United States that are caused by obesity (Allison et al.). If one were to read the article, they would find that the authors note, "our calculations assume that all (controlling for age, sex, and smoking) excess mortality in obese people is due to obesity" (1536). This means that every death of a fat person was attributed to obesity.[1] We also cover such topics as the science news cycle (Chan) and the conflation of weight and health (Ernsberger and Koletsky, 223). It is usually during this part of the workshop that people begin to protest. It is often uncomfortable to examine the beliefs that you hold, especially ones that are negative and contribute to the oppression of others. Especially because everyone knows that being fat is unhealthy.

I once had a participant who was angry at my suggestion that fatness did not cause type 2 diabetes. He shared with the group that he knew that fatness caused type 2 diabetes because all of his fat patients were type 2 diabetics. I then asked him if he saw any patients without type 2 diabetes, regardless of size, and he said no—that he only saw individuals with this diagnosis.

What I was trying to point out to him was his own confirmation bias. He believed that fat people got type 2 diabetes, and every fat patient he saw confirmed this for him. He failed to consider, however, that many of his patients with type 2 diabetes were not fat and that there were many fat people (not his patients) who did not have and will never develop type 2 diabetes.

In the final part of the workshop, I introduce health at every size (HAES), a new medical paradigm that disassociates health from weight and body size (Bacon and Aphramor 5; Bacon et al., "Evaluating" 862; Bacon et al., "Size" 933). I propose ways they may practice HAES in their work and ask for suggestions for ways they believe the HAES paradigm could change the way they approach their practice.

You may be wondering if the work I am doing does any good. I often wonder the same thing. I've yet to undertake an empirical investigation as to whether the workshops affect participants' knowledge of weight and health, change their attitudes about fatness, or influence the way they practice. I like to think that most people leave the space with questions about the dominant discourse around obesity. And I know that, for some, it is a meaningful and life changing experience because I hear from those people in the future. They send an email to thank me for changing their perspective or challenging their colleagues' perceptions.

I believe that raising consciousness is always a positive endeavour. Whether this is done by blogging (Read), providing resources to marginalized communities ("Nalgona Positivity Pride"), synchronized swimming (Aquaporko), or publishing (Lee 11), it all refutes the normative understanding of fatness and fat embodiment. Those of us involved in this work know that it isn't easy and that the backlash can be severe. At a conference in 2010, Michael Gard and Paul Campos presented their evidence that the obesity epidemic was a social construction and that the relationship between weight and health was not as clear cut as often suggested at a conference in 2010. Towards the end of the session, a man stood up in the middle of the room and exclaimed, "I have never seen a fat person hike the Abel Tasman."[2] The room fell silent, as his unspoken accusations settled around us. Fat people are lazy, inactive.

I couldn't help but sit straighter in my chair and announce in kind, "Well, I've never seen a man load a dishwasher." The room filled with guffaws and laughter while he slowly took his seat with a confused expression. I don't think he understood the logical fallacy we were both making, but it may have reinforced it to others present. Most importantly, I wasn't about to let his "everyone knows this to be true!" privilege-based statement go unchallenged.

We do a disservice if we assume that people aren't willing to listen, learn, or be reflective on their own beliefs and behaviors. Many are. And in my workshops, the dissenters, those who are not willing to engage with the material at all, are few and far between. The work of educating the public about issues related to fat activism, fatness and health, and weight discrimination will continue to be an important task for those up to the challenge. Recently, my workshops have changed in tone. I am less focused on educating those in attendance on the science and untruths that are rampant (although I do still cover them briefly) and more focused on ethics. What is the ethical practice of those in healthcare (and other service professions) in providing care for fat patients? If we know that weight loss is unsuccessful for 95 per cent of those who attempt it, how is it ethical to put this forth as a medical prescription or therapy goal? Even if being fat is the unhealthiest thing in the world (which it most certainly is not), does that make it okay to shame and discriminate against fat kids in educational settings? These are the themes that centre my workshops now.

The stigma and discrimination that fat people face are "key social and environmental factors that contribute to health" (Greenberg et al. 1342). It is not just medical care providers that need to unpack their attitudes about fatness—its teachers, social workers, and government officials. It's everyone.

Endnotes

1. Fat activists have been asking for decades, "How old does a fat person have to be to get to die of natural causes?"
2. The Abel Tasman is a popular hiking trail on the South Island of Aotearoa, New Zealand.

Works Cited

Adams, Kelly, M., et al. "The State of Nutrition Education at US Medical Schools." *Journal of Biomedical Education*, vol. 2015, 2015, pp. 1-7.

Allison, David B., et al. "Annual Deaths Attributable to Obesity in the United States." *Jama*, vol. 282, no.16, 1999, pp. 1530-38.

Amy, Nancy K., et al. "Barriers to Routine Gynecological Cancer Screening for White and African-American Obese Women." *International Journal of Obesity*, vol. 30, no. 1, 2006, pp. 147-55.

Aquaporko! *Aquaporko! The Documentary*, 2013, aquaporkofilm.com/. Accessed 7 Feb. 2016.

Bacon, Linda, and Lucy Aphramor. "Weight Science: Evaluating the Evidence for a Paradigm Shift." *Nutrition Journal*, vol. 10, no. 1, 2011, p. 69.

Bacon, Linda, et al. "Size Acceptance and Intuitive Eating Improve Health for Obese, Female Chronic Dieters." *Journal of the American Dietetic Association*, vol. 105, no. 6, 2005, pp. 929-36.

Bacon, Linda, et al. "Evaluating a 'Non-Diet' Wellness Intervention for Improvement of Metabolic Fitness, Psychological Well-Being and Eating and Activity Behaviors." *International Journal of Obesity*, vol. 26, 2002, pp. 854-65.

Bocquier, Aurélie, et al. "Overweight and Obesity: Knowledge, Attitudes, and Practices of General Practitioners in France." *Obesity Research*, vol. 13, no. 4, 2005, pp. 787-95.

Budd, Geraldine M., et al. "Health Care Professionals' Attitudes about Obesity: An Integrative Review." *Applied Nursing Research*, vol. 24, no. 3, 2011, pp. 127-37.

Campos, Paul, et al. "The Epidemiology of Overweight and Obesity: Public Health Crisis or Moral Panic?" *International Journal of Epidemiology*, vol. 35, no. 1, 2006, pp. 55-60.

Campos, Paul. *The Diet Myth: Why America's Obsession with Weight Is Hazardous to Your Health*. Gotham, 2005.

Carryer, Jenny. "Embodied Largeness: A Significant Women's Health Issue." *Nursing Inquiry*, vol. 8, no. 2, 2001, pp. 90-97.

Chan, J. "The Science News Cycle." *PhD Comics*, 2009, www.phdcomics.com/comics.php?f=1174. Accessed 7 Feb. 2016.

Cramer, Phebe, and Tiffany Steinwert. "Thin Is Good, Fat Is Bad: How Early Does It Begin?" *Journal of Applied Developmental Psychology*, vol. 19, no. 3, 1998, pp. 429-51.

Crandall, Christian, and Monica Biernat. "The Ideology of Anti Fat Attitudes." *Journal of Applied Social Psychology*, vol. 20, no. 3, 1990, pp. 227-43.

Drury, Alegria, et al. "Exploring the Association between Body Weight, Stigma of Obesity, and Health Care Avoidance." *Journal of the American Academy of Nurse Practitioners*, vol. 14, no. 12, 2002, pp. 554-61.

Ernsberger, Paul, and Richard J. Koletsky. "Biomedical Rationale for a Wellness Approach to Obesity: An Alternative to a Focus on Weight Loss." *Journal of Social Issues*, vol. 55, no. 2, 1999, pp. 221-60.

Foster, Gary D., et al. "Primary Care Physicians' Attitudes about Obesity and Its Treatment." *Obesity Research*, vol. 11, no. 10, 2003, pp. 1168-77.

Gard, Michael. *The End of the Obesity Epidemic*. Routledge, 2011.

Greenberg, Bradley S., et al. "Portrayals of Overweight and Obese Individuals on Commercial Television." *American Journal of Public Health*, vol. 93, no. 8, 2003. pp. 1342-48.

Hague, Anne L., and Adrienne A. White. "Web-Based Intervention for Changing Attitudes of Obesity among Current and Future Teachers." *Journal of Nutrition Education and Behavior,* vol. 37, no. 2, 2005, pp. 58-66.

Jutel, Annemarie. "Weighing Health: The Moral Burden of Obesity." *Social Semiotics*, vol. 15, no. 2, 2005, pp. 113-25.

Jutel, Annemarie. "Does Size Really Matter? Weight and Values in Public Health." *Perspectives in Biology and Medicine*, vol. 44, no. 2, 2001, pp. 283-96.

Kelly, Kathleen. *Translating Research into Practice: The Physicians' Perspective*. ProQuest, 2008.

Kristeller, Jean L., and Robert A. Hoerr. "Physician Attitudes toward Managing Obesity: Differences among Six Specialty Groups." *Preventive Medicine*, vol. 26, no. 4, 1997, pp. 542-49.

Maroney, Diane, and Sharon Golub. "Nurses' Attitudes toward Obese Persons and Certain Ethnic Groups." *Perceptual and Motor Skills*, vol. 75, no. 2, 1992, pp. 387-91.

Morrison, Todd G., and Wendy E. O'Connor. "Psychometric Properties of a Scale Measuring Negative Attitudes toward Overweight Individuals." *The Journal of Social Psychology*, vol. 139, no. 4, 1999, pp. 436-45.

Mukohara, Kei, and Mark D. Schwartz. "Electronic Delivery of Research Summaries for Academic Generalist Doctors: A Randomised Trial of an Educational Intervention." *Medical Education*, vol. 39, no. 4, 2005, pp. 402-09.

Nalgona Positivity Pride. www.nalgonapositivitypride.com/. Accessed 7 Feb. 2016.

Pausé, Cat Jeffrey. "Rebel Heart: Performing Fatness Wrong Online." *M/C Journal*, vol. 18, no. 3, 2015, www.journal.media-culture.org.au/index.php/mcjournal/article/viewArticle/977. Accessed 7 Feb. 2016.

Pausé, Cat Jeffrey. "Die Another Day: The Obstacles Facing Fat People in Accessing Quality Healthcare." *Narrative Inquiry in Bioethics*, vol. 4, no. 2, 2014, pp. 135-41.

Pausé, Cat Jeffrey. "X-Static Process: Intersectionality within the Field of Fat Studies." *Fat Studies: An Interdisciplinary Journal of Body Weight and Society*, vol. 3, no. 2, 2014, pp. 80-85.

Persky, Susan, and Collette P. Eccleston. "Medical Student Bias and Care Recommendations for an Obese Versus Non-Obese Virtual Patient. International Journal of Obesity, vol. 35, no. 5 2011, pp. 728-35.

Puhl, Rebecca M., and Chelsea A. Heuer. "Obesity Stigma: Important Considerations for Public Health." *American Journal of Public Health*, vol. 100, no. 6, 2010, pp. 1019-28.

Puhl, Rebecca M., and Chelsea A. Heuer. "The Stigma of Obesity: A Review and Update." *Obesity*, vol. 17, no. 5, 2009, pp. 941-64.

Read, Kath. "Why Do I Have to Keep Saying This?" *Fat Heffalump*, 28 Apr. 2013, fatheffalump.wordpress.com/2013/04/28/why-do-i-have-to-keep-saying-this/. Accessed 7 Feb. 2016.

Teachman, Bethany A., and Kelly D. Brownell. "Implicit Anti-Fat Bias among Health Professionals: Is anyone Immune?" *International Journal of Obesity & Related Metabolic Disorders*, vol. 25, no. 10, 2001, pp. 1525-32.

Wann, Marilyn. "Weight of the Nation Serves Up More Fat-Shaming." *SFWeekly Blogs*, 14 May 2012, www.sfweekly.com/tag/fat-activism/. Accessed 7 Feb. 2016.

26.

"Men Are Not Dogs. They Don't Throw Themselves on the Bones": Fat as Desirable

Victoria Team

Introduction

In Western countries, thinness remains the most privileged type of body and the one most people aspire towards (Grogan). Conversely, fatness is considered ugly, unappealing, and unhealthy (LeBesco). However, in other geographic locations, this culture is different; for example, in Mauritania (Guerrero), rural Jamaica (Sobo), and Ukraine (Bilukha and Utermohlen), women with fuller bodies are considered beautiful. In this work, I share my experiences of being slim and fat, my perception of ugliness and beauty, my feelings of being not in the right body and in the right one, and my initial dissatisfaction and later satisfaction with my body image. My autoethnographic exploration of thinness relates to the period of my adolescence and young adulthood and is limited to the country of my birth, Ukraine. I explore fatness as my midlife experience in Australia. I further examine the interrelations between body image, gender, age and culture in historical and geographical contexts.

Not in My Skin

In Ukrainian culture, from the mid-1960s to early 1980s, fat and curvy women were considered beautiful, and attractiveness was not linked to thinness (Bilukha and Utermohlen 132). Slim women looked at fat women with envy. I was tall and slim and, therefore, ugly by Ukrainian standards. For my family, fattening me up was the goal. For breakfast, my mum would cook me semolina with full-cream milk, adding butter, egg yolk, and chocolate for good measure. I was told to not run a lot and to lie down so that the "fat gets collected," as she'd say. If I was sent outside, it was because "I needed fresh air to increase my appetite." I was getting vitamins, herbal concoctions, and fresh beer brewers' yeast to receive vital nutrients and to improve my digestion. Taking a teaspoon of fish oil twice a day and drinking a glass of sour cream mixed with beer were two of my mum's worst remedies. Although she never forced me to drink them, she would stand there menacingly and watch until I finished. Her silence spoke volumes.

As a child, I would look at Baroque paintings of naked female bodies in art books and encyclopedias with such envy. Women's bodies in Rubens's paintings were my beauty ideals. My favourite paintings were *Perseus and Andromeda* and *The Three Graces*. I also admired the limbless body of Venus de Milo and the headless body of Nicki Samothrakis. The body shape was obviously much more important to me at that time than having my arms and brain. My stepfather was a professional painter. I would pose for him for hours hoping to see the image of one of the beautiful Greek goddesses. However, to my dissatisfaction, I always saw sketches of a skinny girl in a loose fit polka-dot pajama dress looking back at me. I would then cry and run to my grandma, complaining he'd painted an ugly picture of me.

I had even more troubles in adolescence. My grandfather would repeatedly offer me the following Ukrainian proverb about my weight: "Men are not dogs; they don't throw themselves on the bones." Negative comments made by male family members can be very influential (see McCabe and Ricciardelli). He would urge my mum and my grandma to do something regarding my weight: "Who would want to marry her? She looks as a wooden plank. Who would want to lie with her; it would be the same as to stick your dick through the fence hole." My grandma would reply, "No worries. A customer could be found for any product." Although we were not studying Karl Marx's *Capital* and I knew nothing about the quality of a product and various product values (27), I understood that as a product, I was of poor quality. I hated my body shape; I had a feeling that I was in the wrong body. I was very upset about this error of nature. My grandma would comfort me, saying that men do not just consider body shape when they choose their future wife. Regardless, I was trying to visually improve my shape and give the illusion of a fuller body. I was selecting skirts with folds and pleats. I was wearing five to seven pairs of knickers underneath of my pants to make them look tighter on me. My feeling of being ugly was so intense that I isolated myself, in the same way that fat people do in other cultures (Puhl and Brownell). My mid-life experiences, however, were diametrically opposite.

In My Skin

In my mid-forties, I started gaining weight, sometimes called the "middle-aged spread." Now, in my early 50s, I am fat, I am curvy, and I am voluptuous. Surprisingly, I started receiving frequent compliments from people of all walks of life on the sidewalks and at work. Considering my love of art, the day an artist in Montsalvat, the old art centre in Melbourne, told me, "You are the most beautiful image I've seen here," stuck with me. One of my neighbours, a middle-aged man, noticed my transformation, and started calling me the Beautiful Swan. Whether I was at church or in the park, I was met with people's affirming messages of my beauty and my appeal. I began to wonder why it is now, in perimenopause, that I've received such validating attention? Where was this in my adolescence? It made me reflect on my childhood view, in which curves, fat, and fatness were associated with beauty. It appeared that with my weight gain, I became beautiful. But what is more surprising is that I now live in Australia, where thinness is considered the beauty ideal (Small). In Ukraine, as well, the contemporary notion of beauty as thin has fallen in line with Western trends (Bilukha and Utermohlen). Below, I discuss how I started to love my body and become satisfied with my shape and explain how other factors have shaped my experiences.

Love the Skin You're In

Yes, it is easy to catch phrases, such us "Love the skin you're in" in magazines and makeover shows, and it should be easy to love your skin if you feel that you're in your skin. However, if you don't really feel in your skin or in your right skin, loving it becomes impossible. Body image dissatisfaction and the inability to love one's body can be influenced by parents, peers, and media, as explained by the Tripartite Theory (Thompson et al.). In Ukraine, people were not exposed to Western media, and the local media did not promote thinness (Bilukha and Utermohlen). My beauty ideal was shaped by the images that I saw in my stepfather's art books and by other people's descriptions of what a beautiful body should look like. I did not experience peer pressure directly. I was receiving encouraging comments and suggestions from my peers, such as, "In your case, getting in shape should be really easy—just eat whatever you like and as much as you want." My parents and my grandparents too wished me the best, as all parents and grandparents do. We lived in a collectivist society, and they felt responsible for my body. My body size wasn't appreciated by key members of my family or my culture in general. All of us were at war with my tiny body, and my body was defensive, rejecting all fatty foods. I was losing weight, and we were losing the battle. Loving a substandard and uncontrollable body was impossible.

Now, according to mainstream antifat medical discourse that supports eradicating the so-called obesity epidemic in Australia, I am considered overweight with a body mass index (BMI) of 29; if I add one more kilogram, I would be considered obese. Body image is increasingly constructed by health promotion messages, in which BMI is used as an indicator of change to body mass (Lupton, "How Do You Measure Up?"). However, the accuracy of BMI is questionable (Okorodudu et al.). As a health professional, I understand the importance of introducing some body measurement indices, and as a woman, I realize their labelling power. The problem is with medical discourse that sees fatness as a disease with one solution—weight loss—and all the other myths that operate to oppress and identify fat people as not only ugly in most cases but also unhealthy. As Charlotte Cooper has noted, "It is not the fat body that is an issue, but the cultural production of fatphobia" (1020). In line with the medicalization of fatness, the notion of beauty was replaced with the notion of health, and "fatness becomes a matter of life and death" (Saguy 15). Many women are now experiencing pressure to lose weight for health-related reasons (Lupton, *Fat*), although the benefits and the risks of weight loss are not well-established (Montani, Schutz, and Dulloo) as well as its effects on body image (dis)satisfaction (Gilmartin). Fitspiration is a relatively new social media and lifestyle trend that runs in parallel with healthy weight discourse, and the current requirements for the body are not only thin but also toned (Tiggemann and Zaccardo).

Naomi Wolf in *The Beauty Myth* has discussed the societal pressure on women and girls to comply with the social standards of attractiveness and its potential to grow "so intense that it will become obligatory" (269). What is interesting is that this societal pressure remains the same even if the beauty ideals differ across cultures and change over time. Beauty culture is not static (Anderson-Fye, McClure, and Wilson). Women's bodies too are fluid, as Julia Kristeva argued, and they change across their life stages. Lacking control over their life stages and beauty culture, young women attempt to control their bodies. With time, however, they develop cognitive skills and adopt cognitive strategies that help them to accept their body, which increasingly becomes "socially undesirable" and "largely uncontrollable" as they age (Webster and Tiggemann 249). As an image-concerned child and adolescent, despite having a normal body, I willingly complied with the social standards of attractiveness, which also became my own standards. In my middle age, I willingly reject the societal pressure placed on me regarding my body. I now love my body, and I feel good in my skin. I relate this change to my better cognitive skills that have helped to increase my self-acceptance as well as to older Ukrainian culture, which idealized women's fuller bodies.

Works Cited

Anderson-Fye, Eileen, Stephanie McClure, and Rachel Wilson. "Cultural Similarities and Differences in Eating Disorders." *The Wiley Handbook of Eating Disorders*, edited by Linda Smolak and Michael P. Levine, John Wiley & Sons, Ltd, 2015, pp. 297-311.

Bilukha, Oleg O., and Virginia Utermohlen. "Internalization of Western Standards of Appearance, Body Dissatisfaction and Dieting in Urban Educated Ukrainian Females "*European Eating Disorders Review*, vol. 10, no. 2, 2002, pp. 120-37.

Cooper, Charlotte. "Fat Studies: Mapping the Field." *Sociology Compass*, vol. 4, no. 12, 2010, pp. 1020-34.

Gilmartin, Jo. "Body Image Concerns Amongst Massive Weight Loss Patients." *Journal of Clinical Nursing*, vol. 22, no. 9-10, 2013, pp. 1299-309.

Grogan, Sarah. "Femininity and Body Image: Promoting Positive Body Image in the 'Culture of Slenderness.'" *Contested Bodies of Childhood and Youth*, edited by Kathrin Hörschelmann, Kathrin and Rachel Colls, Palgrave Macmillan UK, 2010, pp. 41-52.

Guerrero, Lindsey A. "The Force-Feeding of Young Girls: Mauritania's Failure to Enforce Preventative Measures and Comply with the Convention on the Elimination of All Forms of Discrimination against Women." *Transnational Law & Contemporary Problems*, vol. 21, no. 3, 2013, pp. 879-910.

Kristeva, Julia. *Powers of Horror: An Essay on Abjection*. Translated by L. S. Roudiez. Columbia University Press, 1982.

LeBesco, Kathleen. *Revolting Bodies?: The Struggle to Redefine Fat Identity*. University of Massachusetts Press, 2004. Print.

Lupton, Deborah. *Fat*. Routledge, 2013.

Lupton, Deborah. "'How Do You Measure Up?' Assumptions about 'Obesity' and Health-Related Behaviors and Beliefs in Two Australian 'Obesity' Prevention Campaigns." *Fat Studies*, vol. 3, no. 1, 2014, pp. 32-44.

McCabe, Marita P, and Lina A Ricciardelli. "Parent, Peer, and Media Influences on Body Image and Strategies to Both Increase and Decrease Body Size among Adolescent Boys and Girls." *Adolescence*, vol. 36, no. 142, 2001, p. 225.

Montani, J. P., Y. Schutz, and A. G. Dulloo. "Dieting and Weight Cycling as Risk Factors for Cardiometabolic Diseases: Who Is Really at Risk?" *Obesity Reviews*, vol. 16, 2015, pp. 7-18.

Okorodudu, D. O., et al. "Diagnostic Performance of Body Mass Index to Identify Obesity as Defined by Body Adiposity: A Systematic Review and Meta-Analysis." *Int J Obes*, vol. 34, no. 5, 2010, pp. 791-99.

Puhl, Rebecca M., and Kelly D. Brownell. "Confronting and Coping with Weight Stigma: An Investigation of Overweight and Obese Adults." *Obesity*, vol. 14, no. 10, 2006, pp. 1802-15.

Small, Jennie. "Women's "Beach Body" in Australian Women's Magazines." *Annals of Tourism Research*, vol. 63, 2017, pp. 23-33.

Sobo, Elisa J. "The Sweetness of Fat: Health, Procreation, and Sociability in Rural Jamaica." *Food and Culture: A Reader*, edited by Carole Counihan, and Penny van Esterik, Rutgers, 1997, pp. 256-71.

Thompson, J. Kevin, et al., eds. *Exacting Beauty: Theory, Assessment, and Treatment of Body Image Disturbance*. American Psychological Association, 1999.

Tiggemann, Marika, and Mia Zaccardo. "'Exercise to Be Fit, Not Skinny': The Effect of Fitspiration Imagery on Women's Body Image." *Body Image*, vol. 15, 2015, pp. 61-67.

Webster, Jessica, and Marika Tiggemann. "The Relationship between Women's Body Satisfaction and Self-Image across the Life Span: The Role of Cognitive Control." *The Journal of Genetic Psychology*, vol. 164, no. 2, 2003, pp. 241-52.

27.

Two Poems

Aries Hines

The Flaps

I pronounce
myself the give-up champion
I give up on apologizing
for my weight with black clothes
old big clothes that never fit
and clothes that say
"don't look at me"

I give up on pretending I need
to be smaller
to smile harder
these delicious criticized layers
warm like a stack of buttered pancakes
thick like a freshly printed manuscript
these are the lips to my rebirth

this
extra thick groove
in my back made to hold
me up when I am
straddling between capitalism
and artistry
femininity and patriarchy

identity and propaganda
spirit and space
crackling at the boiling point of my own insanity

these jagged unabridged flaps
don't answer to anyone they
hold me up from falling
when my anxiety is screaming
and I need the spirits to make
my world quieter
these criticized layers are my wings
and I will use them
to fly through the universe
blowing kisses to morsels of children

raising Black girl identities
with the soul of my pen
allowing them to name

this bridge called my back a sanctuary
the couch they can have
any night of the week
these flaps
the path I point
to ancestors when they need
a fix of the grit in my neck

Weight in Gold

Goddamnit girl
don't you get it yet
you are worth my weight and your own in gold

juggling fear and rejection like back pain

replace lonely with unworthy lovers
look for self-worth in pretty sounding promises

gracious for crumbs or scraps
anything to get you through the tears

you deserve kisses
for every curvature of your quirkiness

you
deserve good love
the kind that stretches into your backbone
elongates down your spine
prickles your neck

flows through your arms and legs
sings in your smile
reverberates when you walk

a love whose melody washes
the memory of all the people who forgot to love you
how low you felt when you lost your job

you are worth my weight and your own in gold
and I say it to you because I don't think you've heard it enough

you heard you were stupid fat or not pretty enough
to reach out into earth for something good

you see love as something to keep away the lonely
I want these words to be your wakeup call

your aha moment
hallelujah holy ghost
fall on the ground and break yourself

I want this to be the moment when all
the confetti and lights rain down on you
as you finally step up for yourself

I want you to break open
transform in new skin
I am praying for your breakthrough
whisper these words over you while you sleep

28.

Being Gentle with Myself: A Lifelong Work in Progress

Stephanie A

This is a story about fear, shame, a major dearth of self-confidence and the discoveries and efforts made to stop playing small from a fat, white, cisgendered, able-bodied, heteroflexible, and middle-class woman with privilege. I acknowledge that my story and struggles are not unique and that there are many other voices who should be lifted and shared ahead of my own, given my privilege. Having been blessed with the opportunity to write for this anthology and recognizing that speaking about my shame and sharing my vulnerabilities is not only part of my healing but may be helpful in some way to someone else, what follows is a snapshot into the past fourteen years of my journey to loving and being kinder to myself.

From as far back as I can remember, I never felt good enough. I always believed that there was something intrinsically wrong with me, which I attributed to being fat, unattractive, and socially awkward. Through messaging from our patriarchal, capitalist culture, my parents (and how they felt about themselves), peers, and Catholic upbringing, I learned that I am not enough—not attractive, smart, funny, thin, interesting, good, fun, talented, assertive, and confident enough. It would be many years later that my older sister told me a truth I had never before considered: "The problem is not that there's something wrong with you; the problem is that you think there's something wrong with you." Beginning in 2004, at twenty-two years old, through exposure to fat fashion groups on LiveJournal and reading books like Marilyn Wann's *Fat!So?* and Margaret Cho's *I'm the One That I Want*, my life began to change as I was exposed to the concepts of body positivity, fat acceptance, and fat activism: a world where all bodies are good bodies, where having a fat body was celebrated, where strangers were working to build each other up, and where I felt at home as a size-eighteen woman.

I'll never forget the moment I read Marilyn Wann's chapter on reclaiming the word "fat"—a word I had learned through social and cultural programming to associate with ugliness, shame, and negativity. She instructs readers to say the "f" word aloud, something I thought was incredibly novel and difficult. Ensuring no one was within earshot, with my face flush and hot, I actually put the book down and whispered the word "fat." I immediately thought "*There's no way I'm going to call myself fat! That would be just opening myself up to criticism.*" I kept trying. I said it over and over again, "I'm fat." Sure enough, I would later learn how right she was: reclaiming the word made me feel more powerful, not more vulnerable. Now, I don't even think twice to use the word as a descriptor of my body, and continue to share with others that fat is not a four letter word when they say "Oh, don't say that about yourself!" or "You're not fat."

Through my mom's modelling of struggles with disordered eating, major fluctuations in weight, and negative self-talk, along with a lifetime of social conditioning and media messaging that fat equals bad, my battle for body acceptance involved me comparing myself to everyone else, belittling myself, and assuming that other people were laughing at me or making comments about my size everywhere I went. The spotlight effect—the tendency to believe you are being noticed more than you really are—was a daily anxiety for me. I spent a lot of time irrationally assuming everyone was negatively evaluating me, when. in reality, most people are so wrapped up in themselves they don't typically notice others.

Through continued exposure to images of diverse bodies in various states of undress online, I was inspired to purchase my first bikini in 2004, which I then tucked away in my drawer like a shameful secret. Vacillating between such thoughts as "Oh no, people are going to see my fatness!" and "Finally, I get to show off my amazing tattoos," in the summer of 2005, I planned a day at the beach with some of my best friends and worked up the courage to bust out my round, bare, hairy, and stretch-marked belly in public. Witnessing my best friend's daughter experience a beach for the first time was glorious and helped reduce my hyperawareness of my exposed flesh. In her book *Wake Up, I'm Fat!*, Camryn Manheim hilariously describes the stress endured by fat people from sitting upright while in a bathing suit. All the rolls fold and gather together, no longer hidden from view as they would be in a vertical or horizontal position. Like her, I performed some shimmying, towel grabbing, and covering manoeuvres in an effort to hide the jelly in my belly. As we left the beach, my flipflops kicked up some sand, and as I was about to apologize to the people behind me, I heard a young woman say, "Did that fat bitch just kick sand on you?" Her friend replied, "Yes! UGH!" Although it stung to receive that negativity and although logically I understood it, since it was not a secret that I am fat, it took time and repeated risks like these to build confidence.

Between 2005 and 2009, I did a lot of things that pushed me outside of my comfort zone and celebrated my fat body and budding self-confidence. I started Gutsy Dame, a small business selling plus-size clothing online and at clothing shows. For the first time in my life, I identified a passion and set a goal: to help empower women on their journey towards self-acceptance through fat fashion. Although the business was short lived, as I didn't believe in myself as an entrepreneur, it was an honour to create something that allowed me to connect with many amazing people, to witness customers lighting up after seeing their reflection in clothing styles and sizes that weren't available elsewhere at the time, and to mirror their own beauty back to them through words of encouragement.

During this four-year period, I also learned how to belly dance without any prior dance training, joined a belly dance troupe, and performed (while terrified) in crop tops at events across Toronto (including Pride and the CNE). Additionally, I had two boudoir photo shoots where I posed in various states of glamour and undress, took burlesque classes through Good for Her, performed burlesque, and won a few stripping contests. I started to experience my body as a tool to express myself and an instrument of pleasure and joy. My fat undulated, jiggled, and bounced as I danced in ways that made me feel proud and beautiful. For the first time, I received admiration, praise, and high-fives from friends, family, and strangers for displaying my fat body. Even though I do not inhabit the more socially acceptable hourglass body type of wide hips, a small waist, large breasts, and a round bum, even though I was still very self-conscious, sucked in my belly, and tried to ensure the most flattering costumes, angles, and positions for my body while performing, never in my life had I experienced the external validation I was now receiving at these events, and it did wonders for me.

I also moved out of my family home in the suburbs to live on my own in Toronto and dated a lot. I considered myself a late bloomer, having my first kiss and becoming sexually active at twenty-one. I spent the next ten years dating online because I was too scared of people rejecting me to my face. Online I was articulate, witty, and attractive, and I put my fatness out there, ensuring others knew what they were getting into by talking to me. Feeling less than whole, I met and often had sex with men through dating sites like Plenty of Fish, OKCupid, and Craigslist, sometimes putting myself in risky situations as I sought validation and worthiness from others.

Starting in high school, I believed that having a boyfriend would make my life better, so in every man I was attracted to, I wondered whether he would be the one to appreciate me, commit to me and show me my worth. Over the years, I found myself in several noncommitted relationships with men who were charming and whom I put on a pedestal, who I fell for hard and fast because they offered me attention and physical intimacy, but who were not interested in being in a committed relationship with me. I settled for less and accepted being treated as though I were disposable because that's what I believed I was worth.

It was only after experiencing a long-term committed relationship between 2013 and 2017 that I clearly saw how desperate I was for love and validation previously and that I had been in love with an illusion I created of these men. When information presented itself that was incongruent with my fantasy of them, I chose to willfully ignore it for the rush of feelings I would get. Since then, I have held that younger version of myself, let her cry on my shoulder, and told her that her worth is not determined by other people. Although ten years seems like a long time to be repeating a pattern, I feel incredibly lucky because some people never heal from self-destructive patterns. Through this relationship, I learned that authentic, healthy love is unconditional, and I am forever changed for having had that experience.

After I ended my relationship in February 2017, I decided to be more social, make new friends, and find folks with common interests. With warm weather coming, I wanted to do something that would get me outside, so I began to entertain the idea of joining a sports team. Outside of gym class and recess in school, I had never played sports in my life. In fact, during tryouts for the volleyball team in elementary school, I threw up after a couple of rounds of a speed-running warm-up and never went back. The story I told myself and bought into over the years was "I'm not athletic. I don't like competition. I'm not fit and therefore shouldn't try." My well-used narrative to describe my fitness to others included "I don't run unless I'm being chased" and "I'm in shape - that shape is round."

After doing some research, I found the Toronto Sport and Social Club offered kickball in spring. Having played that as a kid, I thought "I can kick a big ball rolling slowly toward me and run a base!" Seeing this as the most accessible option for my body, I signed up and my life changed. Playing kickball throughout the spring season allowed me to meet a new group of friends who I became very close with. I loved playing so much I joined a second team through Toronto Kickball League and played with my original team through the summer season as well. Insecurity about my body and fitness level crept in immediately as the topic of signing up for soccer in fall/winter was discussed among my new sports friends. I shared with them that I knew I didn't have the stamina to run the field, that I'd never played soccer before, and that I was intensely afraid of getting hurt. They wanted me to play with them anyway, so with a bit of encouragement, I took the risk. Around the same time, I also joined a one-hour bootcamp led by a personal trainer with a group of older women, all more fit than I.

Through movement and sports:

- I changed my story about my physical abilities from "I can't" to "I'll try" and learned I am not who I've told myself I am all these years;
- My emotional and mental health has improved. I reconnected with the feeling of being naturally high and happy stemming from the rush of endorphins through physical exertion;
- I've become physically stronger at thirty-five than I've ever been. (I catch myself flexing in front of the mirror regularly, excited by the definition that's slowly creeping into my soft arms.);
- I've built confidence and assertiveness that has spilled into other areas of my life, including work and social situations;

- I've learned I can be very competitive during game play but don't care whether we win or lose;
- I've found friends who encourage, support, and coach one another;
- I've felt the beautifully cathartic release of pain and tears many times as I push my body to its physical limits. (I cry often and openly during bootcamp—I have a lot to release!);
- I learned I really enjoy playing sports, and that my fat body is fast and strong. Two things I never imagined about myself;
- I've learned I can be wet, cold, muddy, sore, tired, and very happy;
- I've discovered a drive to want to perform better and feel proud when I try something new; and
- I learned that relying on external motivators and preferring a social element to exercise are not a weakness. (I used to shame myself for joining gyms and then rarely going.). It's just what I prefer.

In the past year, I also stopped eating meat, and my body shape has changed. Over the years, I've come to identify with my fat so much that when I started to see my body was replacing some fat with muscle, I actually worried about how I would navigate the world and questioned what would be attractive or unique about me physically if I became thinner. Through further exploration of meditation and spirituality, I've been reminded that attractiveness comes from how we treat ourselves and others, not from our physical form. I also deleted all my online dating profiles and am choosing to believe that it is possible for me to meet someone offline.

I have good days and days I spend wondering why I'm still making self-harming decisions. At thirty-five, I'm only just now really waking up to how crippling my anxiety and self-defeating thoughts are. And it took feeling like an imposter, crying almost daily, as well as burning out and breaking down over the last four months after receiving a promotion at work to realize it. The disordered eating habits I developed from a young age remain as yet untransformed, and in times of loneliness, stress, anxiety, fear, or exhaustion, I watch too much TV, smoke weed and binge eat to trigger the pleasure centre in my brain and feel grounded. This is something I've always felt great shame about and have only recently started sharing with others. Bringing the shadow sides of ourselves into the light is a crucial step in healing, and talking about it minimizes shame's power.

In the current phase of my journey, my goals are to:

- learn to listen to the wisdom of my heart and body instead of my mind—choosing faith over fear and letting go of anxiety more and more;
- develop a discipline of meditating daily;
- sit with my discomfort—feeling uncomfortable feelings as they arise and supporting myself as though I were holding space for a best friend;
- practice radical honesty and radical vulnerability; and
- find the courage to visualize, dream, and imagine the life I want so the universe can help me create it.

Please remember, our minds can lie, trick and deceive us. It is so good at finding reasons why things won't work out, why it will be too difficult. It throws up obstacles with such ease because it thinks it's protecting us. It can cheat us from taking chances, limiting our potential for growth and discovery of what else is possible. It whispers cold, hard untruths so loud and so often that we cannot help but believe it our whole lives. Question that voice. Whose voice is it? Treat it like your employee and ask it to help you "I hear you and I don't agree. What else is true or possible?" We are not our minds, but the one who observes it. Healing takes a lot of time, trust and work. But what is the alternative? Staying stuck is no longer an option for me. No matter how long it takes. No matter how hard it feels.

Know that you will slip back into old patterns at times, and it is crucial to show yourself compassion; forgive and keep going. Being hard on ourselves keeps us stuck, so I encourage you to make being gentle with yourself a priority in whatever ways that looks like for you. Seek support. Trust the process. Be there for yourself. (Have you ever held yourself, stroked your own arm or face and said, "I'm sorry that you've had such a hard day honey. It's ok. I'm here for you and I love you"?) Be the love of your life. A new reality is being born within us and in the collective. And it begins with love. I don't even know you, and I love you. As poet @yung_pueblo writes, "Your self-love is a medicine for the earth."

Works Cited

Cho, Margaret. *I'm the One That I Want*. Ballantine Books, 2002.

Manheim, Camryn. *Wake up, I'm Fat!* Broadway Books, 2000.

Wann, Marilyn. *Fat! So?: Because You Don't Have to Apologize for Your Size!* Ten Speed Press, 1998.

yung_pueblo. Poem. *Instagram*, November 13, 2017. www.instagram.com/p/BbcNl9XFFP_/. Accessed 19 Oct. 2020.

29.

Interpretation

Jessica Jagdeo

I woke up one morning and rolled over in my bed reaching for my phone. I started to scroll through Instagram more out of habit than interest. A photo of a painting caught my eye with the caption: "I'm feeling this." I was feeling it, too. It was a woman, a fat woman, sitting on a couch with her head back, her legs slightly bent with her feet almost touching, one arm leaning on the arm rest and the other on the back of the couch. Every detail was beautiful. The painting, *Fat Sue*, held the world record for the highest paid painting by a living artist when it was sold for $56 million US ("Lucian Freud").[1]

I don't remember the last time I looked at myself with as much regard as I did that painting. Growing up, my physical appearance became part of my identity. I felt I was open to interpretation. I was too tall, too skinny. Then my "thunder thighs" grew in, so I was told. I developed "child-bearing hips," so I was told. Thankfully I was a "pear shape," so I could dress right for my type, so I was told. I wasn't a girl because I didn't wear skirts, so I was told. With these labels, I saw my reflection.

I put my phone down and went to the bathroom to get ready for work. As I stood in front of the mirror, I raised my shoulders, pushed them back, and they quickly returned to a comfortable slouched position. I turned left, right... ugh this body. I didn't realize that on that day in my self-loathing moment, that painting of *Fat Sue* would force me to face the relationship with myself. I couldn't get the painting out of my head.

I walked to work, and on my way there, I stepped off a curb and instantly felt a shooting pain from my ankle to my hip. "Stupid body!" I stopped. What did I just say? I had enough. Not of my body, but of the way I was treating myself. I decided to see a physiotherapist to help me with my physical pain. I learned the way every part of my body is connected from the brain to the feet. The pain I felt in my ankle, it was coming from an area around my knee—referred or reflective pain. The weeks I had some emotional downs, my body reacted and felt pain. My thoughts were so powerful that they actually affected my body and here I thought that my body was the problem. It was in a way referred pain. It was my self-diagnosis.

My new knowledge sparked an appreciation for the human form, and I made a dedication to love my body, admire it, and explore all the depths of it as I did with that magical piece of art. What if I posed for an artist? Could I learn to undo the years of pain I've carried for so many years? I decided to live the questions and reached out to a professor of visual arts to connect me with an artist. I was ready to pose naked, to expose myself. But then the professor challenged me: "Why don't you do a self-portrait? You are an artist. It doesn't matter if you can paint like Freud, you are up for interpretation." Good point. So, I tried. Line after line, using different mediums and colours, I looked at every part of my body. And you know what happened? Nothing. I didn't just feel better. But I started to reflect on the things I did with my life up to that point, and I felt gratitude. My body had carried my heart and mind through the good and bad without hesitation. I realized that there was more that I needed to do that was critical to my journey than just one night of wine and paint.

Step One: Unlearn—I'm not where I can be. I'm okay with that. I've fallen many times, but I've gotten up many times. I'm proud of that. I'm repeating the same life lessons over (and over and over) again. I'm going to get better at that. But for me, right now, I just need to love myself for all that I am.

Step Two: Learn—I learned the science of my body. I explored the art of my body. I stretched my arms over my head and closed my eyes. As I breathed, I felt my nervous system connected to my brain, my neck, my hips... every inch of me. I couldn't see how I looked. I just felt this surge of life through my body. This is all I have. This body is part of my life. Without it, what could I have done?

Step Three: Keep going—I didn't suddenly start loving my body. But I did stop saying the awful things I would say to myself. I recognize that I will have to continue the practice to be kind to myself. It's true. The way people see me is open to interpretation. For me, my body is an incredible system that simply requires love and care, and it will continue to allow me to live out my dreams. No one else can do that for me, I've told myself.

Works Cited

1. "Lucian Freud Painting of 'Fat Sue' Sells for Over £35m." The Telegraph, 14. 2015, www.telegraph.co.uk/news/newstopics/howaboutthat/11606838/Lucian-Freud-painting-of-Fat-Sue-sells-for-over-35m.html. Accessed 8 Oct. 2020.

30.

We Are the Seeds: Reflections and Conversations on Beauty, Body Image, and Identity with Urban Indigenous Women in Toronto

Emily Claire Blackmoon

Last year, I wrote a small research study (or what they call a "major research part") as part of completing my master's degree in social work at Ryerson University. As a woman of both Indigenous and non-Indigenous descent (I am English, French, and Algonquin, of the Wàwàckeciriniwak or Weskarini First Nation), I knew I wanted to focus on Indigeneity and the effects of colonization in my research.

At the start, it felt like a daunting task. I had never considered myself much of a researcher (or an academic for that matter). I had been working for nearly ten years as a social worker and counsellor in Toronto Indigenous communities. My day-to-day work was talking and sharing, in kitchens and in lodges, around campfires and in groups, with other urban Indigenous women and families. What did I know about research?

For the last decade, my career focused on counselling Native women and girls in Toronto. Despite the "Pocahontas stereotype," as one of my participants put it, of Indigenous women—tall, olive skinned, raven hair, and dark eyed—the majority of girls and women I met and worked with in Toronto were diverse. They were a combination of mixed-racial women, whose nations and communities were long outside the borders of the city. They were Cree-Jamaican girls, who lived in Scarborough, or Vietnamese-Anishnawbe, who attended school in the north parts of Etobicoke. They were Salish mothers, whose home communities were in British Columbia, yet they had spent their whole lives in Toronto and were now raising boisterous and street-savvy city kids. I absolutely love the diversity of Toronto's Native community this way; in many ways, it is so unique. If Toronto is the gateway and meeting point of races, cultures, ethnicities, and orientations, why would the Native community be any different? There are, of course, leaders and members of more local communities, such as the Mississaugas of the New Credit and the thoroughly Haudenosaunee folks from Six Nations. But by and large, the experience I have in working with Toronto Native communities is that we are a tremendous group of diverse First Nations, Inuit, and Métis people. I am blessed to work in this community. I find it comforting, interesting, exciting, and wonderful. Yet it can be challenging in the following ways:

First, like the many Indigenous women I learned and worked with, I too come from a diverse background. I am a woman of mixed non-Indigenous and Indigenous background. I am fair-skinned and grew up middle class in a family that didn't identify with its Indigenous heritage. This allowed me to grow up with undue privileges of both race and class. No one could see I had an Indigenous background. Rather, I was given the free pass of privilege by being seen as a white and middle-class child.

I didn't really explore what it meant to be of Indigenous descent until I went away to university, where I had the opportunity to meet other Indigenous students and faculty and was encouraged by them to reconnect with what was lost. Reconnecting with my Indigenous ancestry became an act of reattaching a bloodline once suffocated and suppressed beneath the colonial family narrative of whiteness. As one of my great teachers, Indigenous scholar Dr. Cyndy Baskin, writes, when it comes to both Indigeneity and social work, I walk as both an "insider and outsider" (28). I have ancestral connections to a community that was obliterated by colonialism, our culture lost through the generations. I see how that disconnectedness haunts my family. Yet I experience all the unearned passes of white privilege This insider-outsider feeling has long created an inner tension within me of whether or not I belong in the community, or at ceremony, and whether the work I do as a social worker is ever good enough or traditional enough. It has made me question whether I am, or ever could be (as both a person and a social worker), "Native enough."

Body Politics

Issues of identity and looks were often hand in hand in our therapeutic narratives. I found myself sitting with many young Native women who were bullied for their weight, who struggled with depression, or who would cut when they felt anxious in public or at school. They talked about being cyberbullied, being stressed out taking "the perfect selfie," being teased for being two spirited and wearing "men's" clothes, or being told that they weren't Native enough by members of their own communities. This violence, literal and otherwise, was a brutal attack against their souls and bodies.

I am thirty-six years old and a woman now. But as a child and youth, I was taunted for my weight and struggled with bulimia and dysfunctional eating patterns for years. From the insults of being called "dogface" or "fat ass" by other kids, to threats of physical and sexual violence by one particularly aggressive bully, to the passing commentary of well-meaning relatives stating "You could be pretty if you just lost some weight," and to the sexual violence I encountered in my teens, my self-esteem in my own body and beauty was abysmally low. By the time I entered university, my self-worth was nearly obsolete.

But then, I started to learn about my history, tradition, and culture. When I did this, it was then that my body and my soul, in connection, began to heal. I began to feel beautiful.

The research I conducted in the spring of 2016 centred upon sharing, speaking, and gathering the collective stories of Indigenous women in Toronto and their relationship to beauty. I already know Indigenous women are beautiful, resilient, courageous, and strong. However, given my own disconnection from feeling both beautiful and Indigenous in my formative years, I wanted to know if other Indigenous women in the city had experienced similar things. In this research journey, I spoke with several Indigenous women—urban, many of mixed race, and other diverse members of the community. I was guided by some of the incredible work of Indigenous scholars on urban, mixed-raced Indigeneity, such as Bonita Lawrence and Billie Allan. I began talking with other Indigenous women, with my friends, coworkers, and members in the Toronto urban Indigenous communities. I spoke with Indigenous academics and Elders about some of the reasons why Indigenous women and girls become divorced and alienated from their own bodies, identities, and sense of self-worth. I also asked about the teachings, the knowledge, and the ways of life surrounding our beauty that might have been forgotten? How does an Indigenous woman understand her beauty from the lens of decolonization and in a way that centres Indigenous knowledges?

The conversations were rich. As they sat and shared their stories, we had moments of vibrant laughter and deep reflection. Yet there were also collective acknowledgements of our pain and hardship. We discussed how the Western beauty standard (which is deeply entrenched in colonialism, capitalism, and the patriarchal submission and commodification of the female body) keeps Indigenous women from reconnecting with more traditional, holistic, and community-based ways of expressing beauty. A Toronto-based Cree Elder told me about how early photography of Indigenous women showed that many women from different nations were adorned with beautiful textiles, beadwork, skins, and face makeup. She explained that this wasn't for vanity or for sexual appeal, but for identification; specific patterns, jewellery, and clothes told the story of which nation and community a woman came from. Beauty was understood as the holistic way a woman led her life—whether or not she was a good community member, a good helper, a good leader, a good healer, a good sister, daughter, partner, or mother, and whether or not she lived her life fully and with meaning. Thus, modern day concepts of beauty and aesthetics are a colonial tool that separate Indigenous women from traditional understandings of beauty (Blackmoon 11)

In the sharing circle, participants discussed how they navigated their mixed Indigenous identities in a large urban sprawl and how the mainstream, Western narratives of beauty had affected their own sense of identity and self-esteem. One participant discussed how she couldn't live up to that "Pocahontas" standard of what Indigenous women are supposed to look like. Others discussed a history of eating disorders as well as experiencing feelings of depression or anxiety over their bodies and appearances in their formative years. This changed for many of them, however, when they turned to Indigenous culture in the early adulthood. When asked "What makes you feel beautiful?" participants pointed to family, community gatherings, ceremonies, dancing, activism, and teaching.

One striking note of the conversation centred on how systemic institutions in Toronto inflicted harm upon Indigenous women by virtue of policing and surveillance. One participant discussed how her sense of value and self-worth was affected by the brutality she experienced by the Toronto police; another discussed her ever-present fear of having her Indigenous children removed from her care by the Children's Aid on the sole basis of their Indigeneity. Both women reflected how the brutalization of Indigenous women by state institutions decentred Indigenous women as key, valuable core members of their communities and, in essence, made them feel ugly and unwanted (Blackmoon 31-39)

Similar research studies have noted that the more a young person is centred in their culture, the less affected they are by external measures of attractiveness and self-worth (Schooler and Daniels 11-18). At nineteen, I stumbled into the Aboriginal Students Centre at my university, curious and wanting to know about that part of my family's ancestry, which felt lost and silenced. Being able to walk in community, being in ceremony, and being accountable to myself and to others as a person of Indigenous ancestry have made me feel beautiful. Walking out of the sweat lodge, or cleaning up the dinner dishes after running a community group, or sitting with a youth in my office, or talking about their lives—this makes me feel very beautiful. When Indigenous women (trans and two spirit included) are centred in the community—be it the urban Indigenous community or the larger urban community of Toronto—their worth, value, and beauty are affirmed. This buffers against external measures of aesthetic and surface standards of beauty or prettiness. When considering our beauty, our teachings ask us to find our value by digging deep into who we are and what we do for our communities, families, ancestors and the generations to come. In honouring them, we honour ourselves, and, thus, we are beautiful.

Gimikwenden ina? Do You Remember?

Recently, I had a dream. I was sitting in a large circle with my Anishnawbe ancestors, all women. They were talking to one another and passing along a large apple. Each woman took a big bite of the apple and then passed it to the next. When the apple came to me, there was only a core left. I started to cry. "You didn't leave any for me. There's none left." "Don't be so ungrateful," said one of the grandmothers tersely, "There's still a bit there. And we have left you the seeds." Many Anishnawbe Elders teach that the memories of our families are carried downstream, through the generations, living forever in our blood.

Our Medicine Wheel teachings tell us about the interconnection of spirit, emotion, mind and body. The Medicine Wheel represents many things and has many interpretations, depending on the nation and the person who is teaching it. In the teachings I have received (from predominantly Haudenosaunee and Cree Elders who teach in Toronto), the Medicine Wheel represents the aspects of person and our true nature as holistic beings. To be in balance is to be right with all four directions of the wheel. This is how I now understand beauty as well—by working to heal my spiritual, emotional, cognitive, and physical wounds. By planting the seeds of my bloodline into working for, and with, the urban Toronto Indigenous communities, I strive to honour my ancestors, my community members, and my body. My beauty comes from working for my community and from walking with my teachings as best as I can. My body is no longer an object for control or commodification, but a vessel by which I can use to support myself and others.

Like many other people of Indigenous ancestry, I am still learning about my ancestry, my community. and my body. This is a journey that I will continue for some time. As Métis teacher Shirley Turcotte explains, from an Indigenous context, healing is not a finite matter with a start and an end; rather, it is lifelong journey. Our work is to walk our path in a good way, with our bodies, minds, hearts, and spirits, in thanks for the life we lead.

I am, I am
In wisdom I walk
In beauty may I walk...
In beauty it is restored
The light, the dawn.
It is morning.

Luci Tapahonso, Navajo

Works Cited

Baskin, Cyndy. *Strong Helpers' Teachings: The Value of Indigenous Knowledges in the Helping Professions*. Canadian Scholars' Press. 2011.

Blackmoon, Emily Claire. *Narratives of Beauty by Indigenous Women in Toronto*. Major Research Paper. Ryerson University. 2016.

Schooler, Deborah, and Elizabeth A. Daniels. "'I Am Not a Skinny Toothpick and Proud of It': Latina Adolescents' Ethnic Identity and Responses to Mainstream Media Images." *Body Image*, vol. 11, no. 1, 2014, pp. 11-18.

Turcotte, Shirley. "Aboriginal Psychotherapy." *YouTube*, 17 Nov. 2012, www.youtube.com/watch?v=MZF5oyn9Avg. Accessed 8 Oct. 2020.

31.

Bowel Blues, Bowel Blows

Jill Andrew

2017. I leave the house stylized, colour coordinated. My complexion beaming. I'm all smiles with the elderly woman who compliments my blazer at the bus stop. My teeth are glistening; my hair is pulled back in a tight ponytail.

I look fabulous. I feel terrible. I'm determined to keep going.

I board the bus.

I need a seat. I can feel the sweat trickling down my armpits—my body's signature reaction to trauma. My stomach is cramping uncontrollably, and my bowels are fighting with me once again.

The seats at the front of the bus are all taken. I don't ask for a seat because I do not 'look' disabled. I am not an aging adult. I am not pregnant. I do not appear sick.

I know better than this. I live with invisible disability and chronic gastrointestinal health issues, but I still catch myself in moments internalizing that particular brand of ableism, ageism, and healthism at its intersection with fatness and Blackness—the kind that leaves you blaming and second guessing the validity of your own embodied experience.

I stand. I stand for the entire ride.

I get to the subway, and I feel wonderful.

The cramps have stopped. I'm on with my day. No more profuse sweating. The feeling of the proverbial knife stabbing me from my inner navel out has subsided. I congratulate myself for leaving the house, for performing a 'good' body and for not being 'trapped' by my body for yet another day—an absurd toast to neoliberalism and boot strap ideology.

"Mind over matter"—another dangerous dualism we've been socialized to believe. It has gotten me through yet another moment—another moment of ignoring my pain, ignoring myself, leaning into denial, latching on to 'self-help' and forcing myself to perform "normal," "healthy," and "productive" on the move. This is a key exaggeration that often masks the exasperation of anxiety, of not knowingness—that gain us undue social and cultural capital within our "no pain no gain," capitalist, transactional, and productivity-obsessed society.

I exit at Bloor and Yonge, and then it happens...

[LOUD BOWEL SOUNDS]

BBBBBBBBBBBBBBBBBFFFFFFFFFFFFFFFFFFFFFFFFFFFFF COCOCOCOTATATA

BBBBBBBBBBBBBBBBBBFFFFFFFFFFFFFFFFFFFFBBBBBBBBB BB BBBBBBBFFFFCOCOCOCOTATATA

An EPIC explosion!!!!!!!!!!!!!!!!!!!!!!

I stand there EXPOSED.

I stand there SOILED.

I stand there ALONE.

I stand there ALONE in a packed subway station.

I stand there stylized, colour coordinated. My complexion beaming.

I stand there in the stench—a painful reminder of how powerful my body is, how deliberate she can be, how powerful we are, how deliberate we can be, how powerful I am, and how deliberate I can be. Control is never absolute. Matter in mind, mind in matter.

I stand there in the stench. My body is reminding me that I should always listen to her—trust my gut (pun intended)—that I should not push myself beyond my limits and that there is no gold star for running someone else's race.

I stand there in that stench until the shock wears off. Have I really just pooped my pants in public? Has anyone noticed? Do I smell? In a moment of dissociative desperation, I think back to being a kid. If I close my eyes, maybe I'll just disappear.

The day before, I had been editing my dissertation and reading Julia Kristeva's Powers of Horror. I had ended near a reflection on abject theory, the abject. I was making linkages between this theory and the praxis of surviving anti-fatness and anti-Blackness, of living while fat and Black. I am standing at Bloor and Yonge in horror and feeling anything but powerful.

I burst into laughter—a LAUGH I cannot control—a laugh that has undoubtedly called attention to myself. I stop abruptly. I worry it may soon turn to tears. It does. My tears reconcile the reality of my body.

A good night's sleep is a celebration. It's often a complex dance between slumber and fullness, discomfort, bloating, that stabbing feeling from the inside out, backed up, back pain, and stomach distention. I urinate frequently through the night due to constipation and its added strain on my bladder and my pelvic floor muscles.

At first, I stop at 9:00 p.m., then I try 8:00 p.m., then 7, then 5. It's now midnight, and I'm thirsty. I swallow my own saliva. When you don't sleep well, it means you can't function to your fullest potential. Sure, it's common sense, but in a faulty world where all too often we are only judged by our last achievement, the grip of perfection holds tight.

I forget that our bodies are entwined in processes of becoming—being made and unmade through movements and connections with other beings and things—rather than as separate fixed or stable units of matter (Helps 130).

I am in pain but also weirdly entertained by the random theoretical connections I'm trying to make while in soiled pants. Goodness, can we never take a break from productivity?

Black womxn feel pain. Black fat womxn feel pain. We also feel great joy and satisfaction.

We feel. Our bodies remember. Our bodies hold complex memories: "To be an embodied Black woman is [also] to know joy, subjectivity, pleasure and the latent capacity to enjoy being seen: to, in a sense, transcend invisibility and to resist erasure" (Melancon and Braxton ix).

I am strong but neither my strength, my sartorial choices, nor my melanin inoculate me from hurt. It is impossible to fully escape the matrix—the interlocking tensions of inequity. Today, I'm literally reeking in it.

Despite my resilience, humour, accommodation, and resistance as a Black queer fat woman, when my humanity is ignored, questioned, or trivialized it can and does hurt that much.

I make my way upstairs and get to a washroom. I make no eye contact. I clean myself the very best I can inside the tiny washroom stall. It is not perfect.

I ready myself for the journey home.

I think about taking a cab at this point, possibly having to ride with the windows down, but then for some reason, I realize I need to journey back as I came. It's cathartic, or maybe it's self-deprecating. I'm not sure.

I must remember this day forever.

Constella.

Resotran.

Glycerin Suppositories.

Stool Softeners.

Senokot/Senna Laxatives.

Tylenol 3.

Oxy.

Colyte.

RestoraLAX.

Lactulose.

Metamucil.

Benefibre.

Yoga.

I think about all of these, my hospitalizations, the close calls, my bowel obstructions and my surgeries.

I stand on the subway for several stops.

It's now time to board the bus invisibly soiled and fleetingly smelling.

I am stylized, colour coordinated and my complexion is still beaming.

My stomach begins to hurt again.

I need a seat.

This time, I take one.

Commentary

I performed an iteration of this piece on August 25, 2019 at the With/out Pretend Unruly Bodies 3: A Night of Storytelling. With/out Pretend's Unruly Bodies afforded me the opportunity to talk back creatively and with humour against systems, structures, and oppressive narratives that seek to control, discipline, shame, blame, and eject bodies that dislocate the status quo. I was terrified. This was personal, which is precisely why I made the decision to perform. We cannot disaggregate our bodies from the world. Individualizing bodies consequently removes them from the very messy and imbalanced society we live in. It erases the contexts of time, space and place—the very interactions, exhilarating and dystopic, that help shape our bodies. I got to talk about shit—literally. It was most revealing, and I left deeply relieved.

Publicly sharing my story allowed me the space to confront my own internalized stigma. Stigma towards our health is often more debilitating than the health issue itself. People with chronic autoimmune conditions, irritable bowel syndrome, and other related gastrointestinal challenges are often met with public scrutiny, which calls into question their health status. The social meanings attached to some bodies tend to become internalized and exert a powerful influence on an individual's sense of self, feelings, and inner worth (Shilling 73). When fleshy bodies are discredited for not measuring up to people's expectations, especially those who wield significant power within our families, social, and career circles or within the institutions we are perpetually interacting with, the stigmatized individual often internalizes a soiled self-identity (Goffman). People's discrediting beliefs foreshadow discriminatory practices and judgments of one's personal character and performance ability, for instance in the workplace. Not to mention, stigma silences. The journey is often lonely when loved ones and healthcare professionals trivialize or flat out deny health experiences and the negative impact of stigma (Chelvanayagam; Lee and Pausé).

Stigma is exacerbated for fat and Black womxn navigating against the backdrop of anti-Black racism, misogyny, and socioeconomic inequities (Cox), among other intersectional subjectivities and social determinants of health (Raphael). Dr. Onye Nnorom, of the University of Toronto's Dalla Lana School of Public Health, has urged public health officials to recognize racism as a social determinant and to add it to the list of key determinants that help or hinder health outcomes (Goffin). Furthermore, the impact of "weathering"—as a way of explaining the toll of discrimination and inequitable access to resources on Black womxn's health outcomes—cannot be dismissed (Geronimus).

Fat bodies are framed as uncanny, excessive, and literally bursting out of bounds (Braziel and LeBesco). Similar to the framing of Black bodies (hooks; Luckett; Shaw), fat bodies have been socially constructed as out of control, lacking self-determination, and are often painted as an unhealthy menace to health care (Ellison, McPhail, and Mitchinson; Saguy). This, even as scientific research continues to demonstrate the flawed basis of body mass index metrics and DSM-V narratives of 'obesity' as indicators of health (Bacon; Bacon and Aphramor) and exposes the fatphobia and racism within the very biopedagogies—the overt and hidden curricular teachings about bodies and health that become the basis of biomedical rules constructed to essentially govern, regulate, and categorize bodies. It is significant to note that these processes of pathologizing and stigmatizing fat Black women's bodies are interlocked in histories of colonialism, scientific racism, and the conflation of fatness and Blackness with moral and aesthetic inferiority (Strings).

Fat stigma intersects with "controlling images" (Collins) of Black women to lay bare what Andrea Shaw argues is the particularly provocative way in which fatness and Blackness intersect. According to Shaw, "Fatness is an evocation of blackness because contemporary western culture understands the fat body as denoting what the Black body was always thought to signify: bodily indiscipline and rebellion" (Shaw 143). Similarly, Kathleen LeBesco argues, "The stigma of fat clusters around the stigma of poverty and non-whiteness with the effect of depriving individuals of their rights as citizens" (63).

Kelly Hoffman et al. describe how as a result of racial bias in the medical treatment of African American people, pain concerns are more likely to be ignored, and they are often denied less intrusive options because of racist assumptions pertaining to their pain threshold relative to white patients. A racist assumption of biological difference is at the heart of this. Similar research has indicated differential treatment between people labelled as 'obese' and those who are perceived as thin or at 'healthy' weights, whereas fat people were more likely to be judged as immoral, blamed for their weight, and were less likely to receive necessary care (Lee and Pausé). I experienced this personally in part of my body story that precipitated "Bowel Blues, Bowel Blows:"

In the early fall of 2016, I receive emergency surgery for another high-grade bowel obstruction. On the day of my surgery, my surgeon tells me I am obese and cautions that because of my fat stomach, infection is imminent. I ask her pointedly if thin people ever got infected. She reiterates my size. She doubles down. I ask her about various less intrusive treatment options and surgical methods. Again, she reminds me of my weight and tells me she has nineteen years of experience, so she knows best. I'm still talking, but she's practically out the door.

In the moment I ponder, "What about the thirty-plus years of experience I've had in and with my own body?" Is it now irrelevant? *I wonder if my attire—the worn, black "trashy" track pants, night shirt, and ratty sweater I put on in the mad dash to the hospital—may be colouring the condescending treatment I'm receiving. Would a suit have made a difference? Or maybe it's simply the postal code? Or maybe I should mention my doctoral candidacy? Or maybe I should just place a bag over my head so I'm faceless.*

In the surgical suite as we wait for the anesthesiologist, the surgeon and members of her team proceed to talk about their lazy, 'obese' pets. I lay conscious and fat on the surgical table with my stomach exposed feeling pain but doing relatively okay thanks to the ER morphine drip. I state that my own cat had been labelled 'obese' by my vet, but I tell them I have a "health at every size" cat who is anything but lazy. They don't get it. They look at me as though I speak gibberish.

The day of my discharge my surgeon discovers my incision is infected. Self-fulfilling prophecy maybe? She proceeds to use a pair of surgical scissors she pulled from her white coat—not from a sterilized tray or solution—and partially opens my wound without any anesthesia, and it kills! She says opening is necessary to aid the healing process. I scream. I scream. I scream. She looks at me, puzzled and says, "It doesn't hurt that much." I am in shock and sheer disbelief. She continues. I continue to scream, and then I stop. My tears simply ran from my right eye to the side of my cheek then into my ears. My incision is redressed. I am discharged.

I continue to live with the mental and physical residue of this ordeal. Fashion, dress, and personal style are integral to how we prepare to engage in the outside world (Abellar; Entwistle; Rocamora; Smelik and Woodward). They help (re)present us while also making us present. I sometimes find myself engaged in extensive impression management and a – "triple consciousness" of my corporeality... size, gender and race – contemplating what to wear to medical appointments and how my sartorial choices may be (mis)interpreted and stereotyped.

I never forgot the surgeon's response as she proceeded to explore my incision. "*It doesn't hurt that much*" she said in an aloof manner. It did, and it still does. I reflect on the various violences Black womxn often face, the accommodations and the resistances we consistently undertake, and the pain of having our lived experiences questioned, minimized or otherwise erased. Fat Black womxn who dare to be bold, opinionated, and difficult, who ask too many questions and demand accountability especially from those with authority, and who take up plenty space in with and through our fleshy bodies are exactly what we need in place.

Works Cited

Andrew, Jill. "Foreword: A Little Fatshion Note on the Power of Clothing." *The Little Book of Big Babes*, edited by Rachelle Abellar, Archive Six, 2015, pp. 1-3.

Cox, Joy Arlene Renee. *Fat Girls in Black Bodies: Creating Communities of Our Own*. North Atlantic Books, 2020.

Bacon, Lindo. *Health at Every Size: The Surprising Truth about Your Weight*. Benbella Books, 2010.

Bacon, Lindo, and Lucy Aphramor. "Weight Science: Evaluating the Evidence for a Paradigm Shift." *Nutritional Journal*, vol. 10, no. 9, 2011, pp. 1-13.

Bacon, Lindo, and Lucy Aphramor. *Body Respect: What Conventional Health Books Get Wrong, Leave Out, and Just Plain Fail to Understand about Weight*. Benbella Books, 2014.

Braziel, Jana Evans, and Kathleen LeBesco. *Bodies Out of Bounds: Fatness & Transgression*. University of California Press, 2001.

Chelvanayagam, Sonya. "Stigma, Taboos and Altered Bowel Function." *Gastrointestinal Nursing*, vol. 12, no. 1, 2014. *MAG Online Library*, https://doi.org/10.12968/gasn.2014.12.1.16. Accessed 8 Oct. 2020.

Collins, Patricia Hill. *Black Feminist Thought: Knowledge, Consciousness and the Politics of Empowerment*. 2nd ed. Routledge Classics, 2009.

Ellison, Jenny, et al. *Obesity in Canada: Critical Perspectives*. University of Toronto Press, 2016.

Entwistle, Joanne. *The Fashioned Body: Fashion, Dress & Modern Social Theory*. 2nd ed. Polity Press, 2015.

Geronimus Arline T. "Understanding and Eliminating Racial Inequalities in Women's Health in the United States: The Role of the Weathering Conceptual Framework." *Journal of the American Medical Women's Association*, vol. 56, no. 4, 2001, pp. 133-50.

Goffin, Peter. "Effects of Racism on Physical Health Should be Tracked, Says U of T Doctor." *Toronto Star*, 21 Feb. 2017, www.thestar.com/news/gta/2017/02/21/effects-of-racism-on-physical-health-should-be-better-tracked-says-u-of-t-doctor.html. Accessed 8 Oct. 2020.

Goffman, Erving. *Stigma: Notes on the Management of Spoiled Identity*. Simon and Schuster, 1963.

Helps, Lisa. "Body, Power, Desire: Mapping Canadian Body History." *Journal of Canadian Studies*, vol. 41, no. 1, 2007, pp. 126-150.

Hoffman, Kelly M., et al. "Racial Bias in Pain Assessment and Treatment Recommendations, and False Beliefs of Biological Differences Between Blacks and Whites." *Proceedings of the National Academy of Sciences of the United States of America* (PNAS), vol. 113, no. 16, 2016, pp. 4296-4301.

hooks, bell. *Black Looks: Race, and Representation*. South End Press, 1992.

LeBesco, Kathleen. Revolting Bodies? The Struggle to Redefine Fat Identity. University of Massachusetts Press, 2004.

Lee, Jennifer A, and Cat Pausé. "Stigma in Practice: Barriers to Health for Fat Women." *Frontiers in Psychology*, vol. 7, 2016, https://doi.org/10.3389/fpsyg.2016.02063. Accessed 8 Oct. 2020.

Luckett, Sharrell D. *YoungGiftedandFat: An Autoethnography of Size, Sexuality & Privilege*. Routledge, 2018.

Melancon, Trimiko, and Joanne M. Braxton. *Black Female Sexualities*. Rutgers University Press, 2015.

Rocamora, Agnes, and Anneke Smelik. *Thinking Through Fashion: A Guide to Key Theorists*. I.B. Tauris, 2016.

Raphael, Dennis. *Social Determinants of Health: Canadian Perspectives*. 3rd ed. Canadian Scholars' Press, 2016.

Saguy, Abigail C. *What's Wrong with Fat?* Oxford University Press, 2013.

Shaw, Andrea E. *The Embodiment of Disobedience: Fat Black Women's Unruly Political Bodies*. New York University Press, 2006.

Shaw, Andrea E. *The Fat Black Woman's Unruly Political Body*. Dissertation. The University of Miami, 2004.

scholarlyrepository.miami.edu/dissertations/2198/. Accessed 8 Oct. 2020.

Shilling, Chris. *The Body and Social Theory*. 3rd ed. Sage, 2012.

Strings, Sabrina. *Fearing the Black Body: The Racial Origins of Fat Phobia*. New York University Press, 2019.

Woodward, Sophie. *Why Women Wear What They Wear*. Berg Press, 2007.

Afterword

May Friedman

Several years ago, in response to teasing occurring at my children's elementary school, I found myself giving a talk to a classroom of third graders. Without reference to the fat shaming that had led to my intervention, I went through my usual arguments. Fat people experience oppression in many different ways. Fat occurs for many reasons. Fat does not equal unhealthy. I showed videos and images and welcomed the kids' many questions. At the end of an hour, the children seemed committed to being body positive advocates. The fat shaming ended, and the kids began pointing out examples of fatphobia to one another. Other, more subtle, shifts occurred: children became more mindful of avoiding talking about one another's appearance altogether. One young boy who had refused to take his hat off for six months suddenly became more comfortable with his curly hair and began coming to school bareheaded, explaining that the presentation made him question his own self-talk.

I offer this anecdote not to revel in my own awesomeness but to convey how absurd and how mutable the common-sense notions of fat, body shame, and aesthetics may be. The attitudes in this classroom did not shift because I provided especially compelling evidence but rather because these open eager young people had not yet succumbed completely to the deeply held beliefs about fat people and their bodies that govern our social and political lives. This collection seeks to radically shift the ways we think about fat people and fat bodies by telling our own truths through our own stories. These many stories, of both fat oppression and also fat celebration and reclamation, may serve as a travel guide to a new world order—the world that third graders so easily walked into and the world that may seem, to so many of us, mythic and unreachable.

Taking Back Our Space and Making Trouble

My own child, of course, merely rolled her eyes—she's been hearing me preach for years. "When they call me and my friends fat," she said, "I know they mean it as an insult. But I know that it's not true, so I don't really care." Although I stand in awe at her body acceptance, I also marvel at my daughter's ability to use the word fat without flinching. She may not know it, but she's following in a proud tradition, standing on the broad, unapologetic shoulders of fat activists and other size-acceptance advocates who refuse to let the word "fat" sting. The chapters in this collection seek to take the word "fat" and imbue it with new meaning—to reclaim a word that has been degraded and misused. Naming is a radical act. A refusal to succumb to the language of overweight or obesity means also rejecting the judgment and shame that sees fat people as problems to be solved.

And yet—it's not always easy. Within societies that are deeply uncomfortable with and violent towards fat bodies, we may turn that discomfort and violence towards ourselves. The stories in this collection do not shy away from these tender spots but invite readers to shiver in recognition and to look head on at the difficult and messy implications of living in nonnormative bodies in cultures that train us to literally make ourselves disappear.

If naming is a radical act, then merely living in a fat body is a daily radical undertaking, an embodied experience of rejecting the mainstream. The many chapters in this collection aim to make trouble. Although our stories reject most of the mainstream logic about fat folk, we do agree that fat bodies are troublesome, gleefully contesting the normative conventions of mainstream life. We offer our fat bodies and our fat stories as a way of resisting normative logics across our many intersections. We embrace the ways that not fitting, and not fitting in, may expose the narrow limits of societies and communities. Rather, we aim to take up space, literally and figuratively. We use our big bodies, and we use our words here, to stretch—like spandex across a dimpled ass or like a bathing suit that pulls just so—to stretch our understandings beyond what may be considered seemly.

We show that common sense logic may be much more about "common" than "sense"—we know that common sense doesn't offer much that's sensible. This collection troubles fat through many different subjectivities, looking at the specific trouble offered by fat racialized bodies, fat with and as disability, and the mutability of fat across gender and sexual spectrums. We consider the ways that fat literally adds layers to our bodies but also layers in and with our other subjectivities, holding different comfort and pain depending on where, and who, we are. In honouring fat as both a site of oppression and a space of opportunity, we also understand that fat is not flat—it's a complicated and shape shifting experience that may vary body to body and hour to hour.

Where Do We Go from Here?

Although reams of words have been written about fat studies and fat scholarship, this collection seeks to take this hard won and critical knowledge and humanize it in order to explore its radical potential. By beginning with embodied stories, *Body Stories* aims to get under our skin and to sit with difficult experiences as evidence of where we have been and where we have the potential to go. We aim to unseat the stories told about us—that we are shameful, dangerous, and out of control—and instead tell our own stories in all their glorious variability. We aim to honour where we are today, amid virulent body hatred, and where we hope to be.

We have a strange hope going forwards, one that is a departure from the expectations of most authors and academics. We hope this book quickly becomes dated. We hope that people will view the violence put towards fat bodies as a historical aberration, with the same quizzical confusion with which we now view the historical persecution of people who are left handed. We hope that the world that the third grade so easily engaged will become our new reality and that the healthist witch hunt that equates obesity with sin and damnation will fade and become merely a puzzling moment in our history.

Of course, although it is our fervent desire to eradicate fat oppression and move to a time where body acceptance and self-love can be taken for granted, we also understand the depth of the challenge and the extent of the work needing to be done. The authors of this collection contribute to the quest to change the world in the name of body integrity and beyond because we acknowledge that our fight for size acceptance is inextricably bound up in other fights. Fat bodies cannot be truly safe until we simultaneously eliminate the impacts of racism, colonization, homophobia and transphobia, violence against people with disabilities, violence against women, and many many other fights beyond.

Ultimately, I hope that my children will have no need to return to the third grade to respond to teasing of their children—that my grandchildren will view this book, and many others, as quaint relics of a bygone time that punished particular bodies, and rewarded others, based on the placement of adipose tissue. Although I understand that this is likely an unrealistic goal, the chapters in this collection give me hope that we are moving toward a just world, one which genuinely acknowledges the beauty and diversity of our embodied positions.

Notes on Contributors

Sam Abel is a social worker and an artist. Her social work practice focuses on refugee settlement, mental health, domestic violence, and fat acceptance. Sam's academic research explores the experiences of fat people in therapy. You can see more of her artistic work @saucy.nudles.

Stephanie A is a lifelong learner passionate about self-healing who believes her purpose in life is to love and be honest, helpful, and compassionate. Currently living and working in Toronto within social services, she cares deeply about seeing an end to all forms of oppression and hopes for the collective healing of all animals (human and nonhuman) and the planet. This is her first published work.

Jill Andrew (she/her) is a child and youth worker, an equity human rights educator and a body justice advocate. Her PhD "Put Together": Black Women's Body Stories in Toronto: (Ad)dressing Identity and the Threads that Bind explores the 'trifecta' of anti-Black racism, sexism and fat hatred experienced by Black women and their accommodation and resistance of dominant body ideals through fashion and dress, activism, self-valuation and social interactions. Jill is the co-founder of Body Confidence Canada and is the Member of Provincial Parliament for Toronto-St.Paul's.

Idil Abdillahi is an assistant professor at Ryerson University.

Emily Blackmoon (French/British/Algonquin) (she/her) is a registered social worker and holistic psychotherapist. She has worked for over ten years as a therapist and case manager specifically within the urban Indigenous community of Toronto, supporting parents, families, children, and youth. In 2014, she completed a four-year training in Gestalt therapy and is now a supervisor. In her therapy practices, Emily combines antiracist, antioppressive, and feminist principals of social work with Gestalt therapy and Indigenous worldviews. Emily completed her master's degree in social work in 2016 at Ryerson

University, focusing her graduate research on narratives of beauty with Indigenous women in Toronto.

Sonja Boon is an award-winning writer, researcher, and teacher. Professor of gender studies at Memorial University, she has research interests in life writing, autoethnography, and feminist theory. Sonja's fourth book, a critical memoir titled, *What the Oceans Remember: Searching for Belonging and Home*, was published in 2019. Twitter @ storied_selves

Carrie Cox is a woman who recovered her life from ED over twelve years ago. She is an activist and advocate who has shared her story in local, provincial, and national media, and has presented at conferences in different parts of the world. Carrie believes in the healing power of stories and is honoured to have her poem, written for her daughter, featured in this anthology.

Liana Di Marco (Liana Guitarbabe) is a super-talented singer, song-writer, poet, short-fiction writer, and artist. All these talents are evident in her book *Beyond Pain—Livin' La Vita*, a powerful, no-holds-barred swipe at pomposity, inefficiency and blatant cruelty in the healthcare system, church hierarchy, child abuse in patriarchal societies, disability advocacy, and other stark injustices tolerated in so-called civilized society. The humour and irrepressible joie d'vivre take the journey "beyond pain to livin' la vita."

Alys Einion is an inclusive feminist academic, author, and expert in reproductive health, rights, and inclusive pedagogies. The founder of Centred Birth Hypnobirthing, she researches and teaches in the areas of gender, reproduction, and sexuality. She is an activist for LGBT+ and gender equality, a goddess-worshipping pagan, vegan, and novelist.

May Friedman's research looks at unstable identities, including bodies that do not conform to traditional racial and national or aesthetic lines. May works at Ryerson University as a faculty member in the School of Social Work and in the Ryerson/York graduate program in communication and culture.

Aries Hines holds an MFA in Poetry from Mills College and a BA in English and African Studies. Her work explores race, identity, queerness, and family. She is currently at work on her memoir and a collection of new poems.

Beatrice M. Hogg is a writer, rock goddess, and social worker in West Sacramento, CA. She has a MFA from Antioch University Los Angeles and a BASW from the University of Pittsburgh. She has over two hundred tee shirts and plans to add more to her collection.

Tierra Hohn, B.PAPM, MPH, is a public health professional, yoga teacher, coach and author. She is passionate about helping other feel comfortable in their own skin and uses her experiences to advocate and build awareness about eating disorders and recovery.

Kelsey Ioannoni is a fat sociologist interested in the politics of the body and body regulation. Specifically, she focuses on the fat body, weight-based politics, and weight-based discrimination. She is interested in exploring the power dynamics between primary care physicians and patients (fat women) and how their conceptualizations of health based on BMI negatively affect the lives of fat Canadian women.

Jessica Jagdeo is a marketing professional by day and creative at every other time of life.

Dorothée Jankuhn (Dot) is a cultural anthropologist turned esthetician and nail tech from Göttingen, Germany. Her life was forever changed when she discovered fat activism and intuitive eating. She now thrives to become Germany's first certified intuitive eating counselor. Dot lives in Berlin, Germany.

Anoop Kaur is a disabled femme writer, healer, animal lover, and food aficionado of Pakistani and Indian descent. Anoop's writing focuses on unearthing and exploring the transformative possibilities of disability justice, self-love, and healing through movement.

Samantha Keene is a lecturer in criminology at Te Herenga Waka—Victoria University of Wellington, New Zealand. Samantha's research interests include critical analyses of gender and gendered bodies, pornography and objectification, rough sex and violence against women. She tweets about these issues via the handle @Miss_Keene.

Crystal Kotow PhD, is a writer, activist, and educator whose research explores fat women's relationships with their bodies. She is a self-identified fat feminist killjoy who practices radical vulnerability in her activism, storytelling, and community building.

Lori Don Levan is an educator and a fat activist/scholar. She is also an active artist/researcher using photography, mixed media, and installation to explore issues concerning the fat female body, corporeality, and beauty. Her work also explores concepts concerning memories lost, found, and the reimagining of personal history. She can be reached at ldlevan@gmail.com.

May Lui is a Chinese and white cisgender woman who is an educator and freelance consultant. She has a master's degree in anti-oppression, and anti-racism education. She is a feminist, activist, accomplice, and general troublemaker for social justice. She describes her body as fat, curvy, and plump.

Cat Pausé, PhD (@FOMNZ) is a fat studies scholar and fat activist in New Zealand. Her scholarship explores the impact of fat stigma on the health of fat people. Her fat positive radio show, Friend of Marilyn, has been on the air since 2011. Find her online today.

Tracy Royce is a fat feminist poet and writer living in Los Angeles. Her work has appeared in *Affilia: Journal of Women and Social Work, The Fat Pedagogy Reader, The Fat Studies Reader, Modern Haiku,* Demeter Press's *Mother of Invention: How Our Mothers Influenced Us as Feminist Academics and Activists,* and elsewhere. Her account of caring for her mother with dementia was recently featured on the "One-Minute Memoir" episode of the *Brevity Podcast.*

Simone Samuels, B.A. (Hons.), LL.B., B.C.L., is a writer, speaker, nonprofit professional, fitness trainer, and content creator. She lives in Toronto, Ontario.

Sucharita Sarkar is associate professor of English at D.T.S.S College of Commerce, Mumbai, India. Her doctoral thesis investigated mothering narratives in contemporary India. Her current research is on intersections of mothers, motherhood, and mothering with body, religion, culture and media. More details of her research may be found at https://mu.academia.edu/SucharitaSarkar.

Christin L. Seher is an associate professor of practice in nutrition and dietetics, codirector of the EX[L] Center for Experiential Education and Civic Engagement and affiliated faculty in Sociology at the University of Akron with research interests in critical food studies, cultural humility training for healthcare professionals, and socialization practices.

Melanie Stone is a PhD candidate in the Department of Women's Studies and Feminist Research at Western University. Stone's dissertation examines the way that mothers with disabilities experience work engagement in London, Ontario. She is also a single mother who teaches disability studies at King's University College and works fulltime as an accessibility specialist.

Leesa Streifler is professor emeritus (visual arts), University of Regina. Her work is in major public collections including the National Gallery of Canada, and the Canada Council Art Bank. She co-authored *Mothering Canada: Interdisciplinary Voices; La maternité au Canada: voix interdisciplinaires* (Demeter Press, 2010). https://www.leesastreifler.com

Allison Taylor is a PhD candidate in the department of Gender, Feminist and Women's Studies at York University. Taylor's dissertation research explores queer fat femmes' experiences of identity and embodiment alongside their strategies for resisting femmephobia and fatphobia in Canadian queer communities, and her research interests include critical femininity studies, queer theory, and fat studies.

Victoria Team, MD, MPH, DrPH, is a research fellow at the School of Nursing and Midwifery at Monash University, and health services research fellow at Monash Partners, Australia. She has been involved in research in women's health and, currently, in the field of wound management.

Judy Verseghy holds an MA from York University in critical disability studies and works as a researcher in in the field of developmental disability. Her academic interests include disability, homelessness, caregiving, motherhood, and fatness. She is a mother of three humans and two cats and loves them all deeply (and widely).

Samantha Walsh is a scholar and activist. She is currently a doctoral candidate at the University of Toronto-OISE In the department of Humanities, Social Sciences, and Social Justice Education (HSSSJE), formerly Sociology and Equity Studies. Her doctoral research is in interpretive sociology with a focus on disability and social inclusion. She holds a master's degree in critical disability studies from York University. Samantha completed her undergraduate degree in sociology at the University of Guelph. She is the director of service at the Independent Living Centre of Waterloo Region.

Liis Windischmann provides women easy ways to live mindfully helping them consciously create happy lives they love with simple ideas to create epic shifts. Her projects inspire people to love and nurture themselves mind, body, and soul. Connect with her on all social media via @liisonlife and at liisonlife.com.

Deepest appreciation to
Demeter's monthly Donors

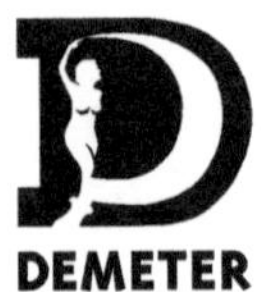

Daughters

Paul Chu
Rebecca Bromwich
Summer Cunningham
Tatjana Takseva
Debbie Byrd
Fiona Green
Tanya Cassidy
Vicki Noble
Bridget Boland
Naomi McPherson
Myrel Chernick

Sisters

Kirsten Goa
Amber Kinser
Nicole Willey
Christine Peets